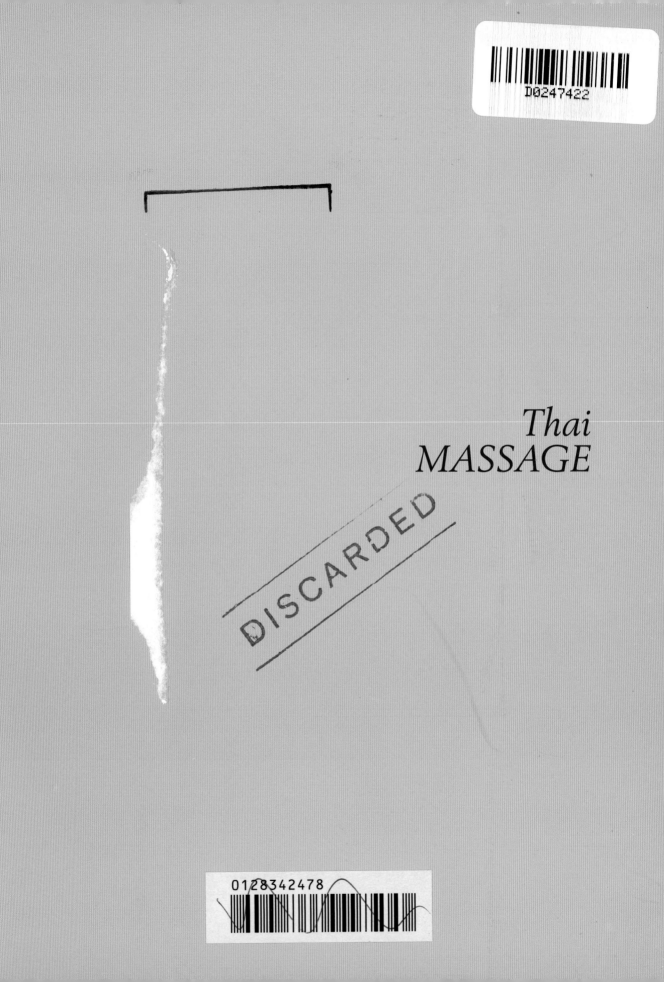

Thai
MASSAGE

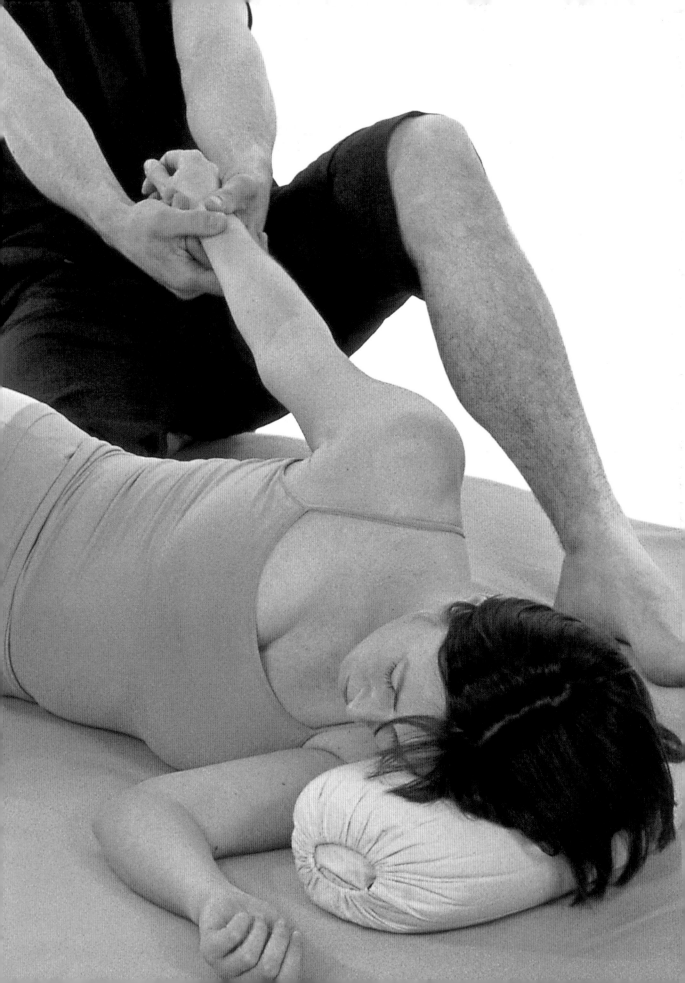

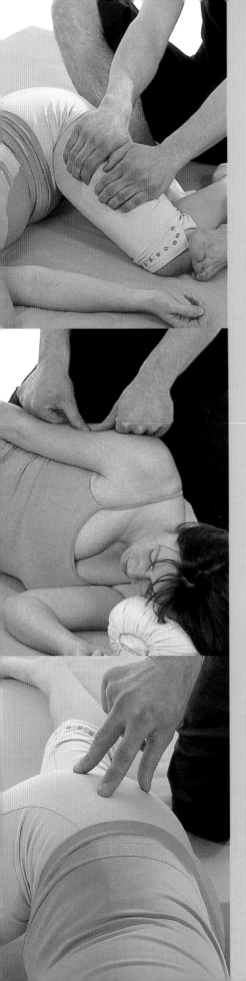

Thai MASSAGE

Niclaire Mann

Eleanor McKenzie

Gaia Books

® This is a Registered Trade Mark of Gaia Books

This edition published in 2005 by Gaia Books
a division of Octopus Publishing Group Ltd
2–4 Heron Quays, London E14 4JP

First published in Great Britain in 2002 as Thai Bodywork by Hamlyn

Copyright © Octopus Publishing Group Ltd 2002, 2005

ISBN 1-85675-241-0
EAN 9 781856 752411

A CIP catalogue record for this book is available from the British Library

Printed and bound in China

10 9 8 7 6 5 4 3 2 1

For further details of the courses and workshops offered by the Devon
School of Thai Bodywork please telephone 01297 32174
or contact Niclaire Mann by email on niclaire@niclaire.freeserve.co.uk

safety note It is advisable to check with your doctor before embarking on
any exercise programme. Thai Bodywork should not be considered a
replacement for professional medical treatment; a physician should be
consulted in all matters relating to health. While the advice and information
in this book is believed to be accurate and the step-by-step instructions
have been devised to avoid strain, neither the publisher nor the author can
accept legal responsibility for any injury or illness sustained while following
the exercises.

contents

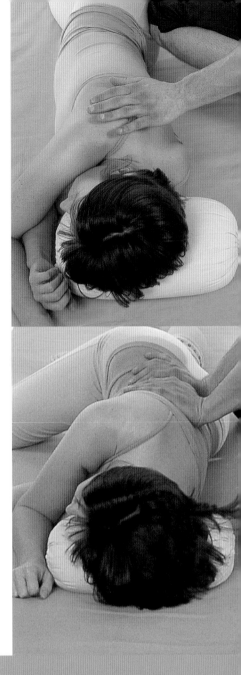

How to use this book

It is important to familiarize yourself with the terminology, basic stances and techniques of Thai Bodywork before you begin. The treatments in this book are arranged according to the position adopted by the receiver: **Supine** (lying on their back), **Side** (lying on their side), **Prone** (lying on their front) and **Seated** (sitting on a mat). Supine is a versatile position as most parts of the receiver's body are accessible. However, some receivers may feel a little shy or vulnerable in supine position if this is their first treatment, so side position is a good alternative. You will find that as your skills develop, you may use up to four positions in any one treatment. With practice you will learn how to move from one position to another using intuition, rather than relying on a set sequence.

Throughout the book, abbreviations are used for the most common techniques such as **Palm Press (PP)** and **Thumb Press (TP)**. Each 'exercise' is illustrated and an arrow (▶▶) indicates at which point in the step-by-step instructions the photograph is taken.

what is thai bodywork?

It is like a thousand gentle waves washing over the body

– Chongkol Setthakorn

Simply put, the main focus of Thai Bodywork is helping to attain or regain 'balance' in the flow of energy (*chi, ki* or *prana*) in the body. It works on both the superficial and deeper fascial layers of muscles, ligaments, joints and connective tissue, and it touches all areas of the body including the nervous, digestive and respiratory systems.

The calming and healing effects of Thai Bodywork on the 'subtle' body have a positive effect on the physical body: it both relieves excess energy and energizes, it is used to maintain wellbeing, and it can also help in the reversal of degenerative conditions.

This ancient art has a close relationship with Indian Ayurveda, yoga, traditional Chinese medicine and Japanese shiatsu. The continuity in the flow of movements, passing through many asana-like sequences (yoga postures) is very similar to Astanga Vinyasa Yoga, while the 'Sen' energy lines which form the backbone of Thai Bodywork are similar in theory to the meridian energy lines in Chinese acupuncture. However, the Sen lines, which are Indian in origin, generally tend to follow the natural form of the body rather than the energy paths of the organs.

origins

The roots of Thai Bodywork lie in Buddhism. When Buddhism spread from India to other parts of Asia, the monks brought their medical practices with them as an integral part of the religious system. Buddhism reached Thailand (formerly Siam) around the 3rd century BC. Where temples were built, medical schools and dispensaries were built adjacent to them and so religion and medicine were as one. Massage and other healing arts were taught in the monasteries and practised within the family. Thus, a two-stranded tradition evolved – written and oral. The written tradition is found in ancient Pali texts. These were the monks' instruction manuals for healing methods and they were kept with the sacred texts of the temple. In 1776, Burma (now Myanmar) invaded Thailand, and many of the ancient Buddhist texts were destroyed. The remaining fragments of the original Pali texts were preserved by King Rama III, who had them collected and inscribed in stone. These stone plaques can still be seen in the walls of Phra Chetaphon Temple in Bangkok, commonly known as Wat Po. The oral tradition was handed down within families, as most people could not read or write. In many respects, it is the oral folk tradition that ensured the continued existence of Thai Bodywork, which would otherwise probably have died out with the destruction of the medical texts.

Dr Shivago

In many ancient traditions, there is often one person who is associated with their foundation: Thai Bodywork is no different. According to the Pali texts, Shivago Komarpaj, a physician and contemporary of Buddha, was the founder of this branch of medicine. There are Thai, Tibetan, Indian and Chinese versions of the story of Dr Shivago. Essentially, Dr Shivago was abandoned after birth, then found and raised by the king. In one account he was born with a bag of acupuncture needles in his hand and was therefore destined to become a doctor, whereas in others, it was simply a skill he chose to learn. Through combining the learning he gained from Atreya, the famous physician and founder of the Ayurvedic system, with his study of a textbook, *The Bodhisattvas of Healing*, Dr Shivago became enlightened as to the nature of all illness. Many regard Dr Shivago as the father of medicine, and practitioners are taught to invoke his spirit in the following prayer before beginning a Thai Bodywork treatment.

thai bodywork today

With the advent of Western medicine in Thailand, traditional Thai Bodywork became neglected. The temples were no longer the centres of education, healing or, indeed, people's social lives. Today this neglect of Thai Bodywork is being reversed. The cost of Western medicine has led to a revival in the art, particularly in rural areas where access to hospitals is limited. Now Thai Bodywork is being used to treat conditions as well as to prevent illness and maintain general health. It is taught throughout Thailand by individual masters and schools, the best known of which, especially for Westerners, are those at Wat Po in Bangkok, and the Foundation of Shivago Komarpaj in Chiang Mai. The techniques and movements in this book are known as the 'northern-style', they are practised throughout Thailand in preference to the 'southern-style', which is known as the 'hard style' and is practised mainly in Bangkok.

prayer

We invite the spirit of our Founder, the Father Doctor Shivago, who comes to us through his saintly life. Please bring us the knowledge of all nature, that this prayer will show us the true medicine of the Universe. In the name of this mantra, we respect your help and pray that through our bodies you will bring wholeness and health to the body of our client.

The Goddess of healing dwells in the heavens high, while mankind stays in the world below. In the name of the Founder, may the heavens be reflected in the earth below so that this healing medicine may encircle the world.

benefits

The uniqueness of Thai Bodywork is its ability to incorporate rather than limit. Its wholesome, rounded flowing style welcomes all to participate. Not just the receiver, but the giver as well comes out feeling more open, stretched, refreshed and 'in balance'. Thai Bodywork achieves this through the application of rhythmic compression to energy lines and points, in synergy with deep stretching movements, gentle rocking and a receptive awareness between giver and receiver to co-create a unique healing experience in the balancing of energies. It is very much like a form of meditation for the giver as both participants move into a space of gentle trust and receptivity, with the receiver being aware of taking part but almost in a trance-like state.

Letting go

Most busy people of the modern world are constantly pushing their bodies with little time for quality relaxation, which is why they need alcohol, cigarettes, sleeping pills, relaxants and drugs to unwind or just to be able to sleep. Thai Bodywork helps to correct this out-of-balance state and enables the receiver to 'let go'. Many people, even fit sportsmen and women, arrive for a treatment 'holding' – holding by shallow breathing, holding tight muscles and holding rigid patterns of thought. The giver creates the right conditions for letting go by encouraging correct breathing, by rocking and by 'giving permission' through supportive touch. A treatment goes on to relieve this 'holding' by gently stretching and lengthening muscles and slowly opening tight joints – knees, ankles, wrists and especially the hips, shoulders and neck. Emotions and holding patterns held in the hara (see page 20) are gently encouraged to unblock, release and let go of unwanted baggage. The large and small intestines, stomach, liver, kidneys, diaphragm and lungs are helped, as the whole body interrelates through the 'chi' connection, whether you have only one, or a series of regular treatments.

If the receiver is able to 'let go' of everyday tension and is relaxed and receptive, this will facilitate a deeper and more positive outcome. Through Thai Bodywork the body is guided to RE-MEMBER with empathy and loving care, to move towards a state of harmony between the physical and the subtle bodies. ALL can benefit. All bodies RE-MEMBER and a number of conditions can be helped, including headache, back pain, sciatica, menstrual pain, irritable bowel syndrome, circulatory problems, respiratory problems, low energy, inflexibility and mobility problems.

Restoring balance

Correcting left-side/right-side imbalance is so important. How many of us stand leaning on a dominant leg? Do you always carry heavy bags to one side? Have you tried brushing your teeth or writing a letter with your other hand recently? The effect of this imbalance travels along the spine and also upsets the left-side/right-side balance through to your toes, finger tips, base of skull and up to your left-side/right-side brain patterns. Thai Bodywork helps the body move back into balance.

A holistic therapy

Even if you have only one regular treatment, with a therapy that provides a whole-body strategy, the benefits are numerous. Every body system is touched on, and while relaxation may be the initial goal, suppleness, improved circulation and organ function, and good mental health are all achievable with Thai Bodywork. In that respect it is a 'one stop shop'. Although other elements of good health such as diet need to be considered, using Thai Bodywork in conjunction with other healthy lifestyle components could considerably simplify the creation of a great body-maintenance package.

giving a treatment

Thai Bodywork is also known as Thai Massage, although in the context of Western practice this can be misleading, as we usually associate 'massage' with a type of tissue manipulation, applied directly to the skin with the receiver lying on a raised bed. Thai Bodywork does include soft-tissue manipulation, but is performed on a mat on the floor with the receiver wearing loose comfortable clothing, preferably of natural fibre. Working on a mat on the floor allows and supports the freedom of movement required for this most wonderful style of work. The giver's own bodyweight, rather than muscular force, is used in the application of pressure to deliver compressions. Stretches and breathing, rocking, relaxing, stretching and working with gravity are equally integral aspects of good treatment. Most importantly, the practitioner's attitude and approach – working from a place of open heart and compassion – is as essential as good technique.

The quality of treatment comes from the carefully tuned 'listening skills' and experienced quality of touch from the giver together with good technique and practice. A traditional Thai Bodywork giver needs to trust in her or his intuition, rather than the structured diagnosis used in various other disciplines, which can often get in the way as the body reacts and changes to every touch.

On a practical level, there are a few simple guidelines that you should always follow:

1 The giver should always check the medical history (past and present) of the receiver to help them with their approach to treatment. If there is any doubt about an illness, condition or injury, ask the receiver to refer to their doctor for advice. (See also, When to take care, right).

2 No matter how many times you have treated a person, never assume you know their body, as our bodies are in a state of constant change on many levels.

3 The room you use for treatment should be warm and well aired.

4 The receiver should not eat for at least 1½ hours before a session.

5 Before 'stepping into' the receiver's space, the giver should close their eyes, breathe deeply and take their time, allowing only thoughts about the treatment to enter their mind.

6 If the giver feels uncomfortable about giving a treatment (for whatever reason), they should wait until they feel more positive.

7 The duration of a treatment is the choice of the receiver – it could be anything from half an hour to 3 hours. Generally speaking, 2 hours is ideal, as it allows for a full body treatment and enables both the giver and the receiver to move into a special space of relaxation and meditation.

8 Allow time for the receiver to adjust before getting up after a treatment. Most people feel a little 'spaced out', but in a very nice way! Some people release emotions and feelings that they have never addressed before as a result of treatment. A drink of water and a little time to gain feedback after the session is helpful for the giver and the receiver.

9 Both giver and receiver should warm up before a session by doing a few simple stretches, working on each muscle in turn.

When to take care

As with any therapy there are certain conditions when treatment should not be given.

○ If in doubt about any condition ask the receiver to ask their doctor for approval.

○ Do not work on a receiver who has had recent surgery (within the last three months).

○ For cancer patients, treatment depends on the stage, progression and location of the cancer. Any patient whose cancer is at a vigorous stage needs a doctor's permission before receiving Thai Bodywork. In cases where cancers have been given the all clear or are in remission, Thai Bodywork can be beneficial. If the cancer affects the stomach, liver, spleen or bowels, the patients should not be given hara treatment.

○ If the receiver suffers from high blood pressure, avoid positions such as the Plough where the legs are lifted high over the receiver's body.

○ If the receiver is pregnant, she should avoid Prone position. Hara treatments and thumb press (TP) below the knees and on the trapezius are also to be avoided.

○ Thumb press (TP) should not be performed on varicose veins.

○ If the receiver has suffered a recent injury, for example a twisted knee or ankle, strained lower or mid-back, do not work directly on the area if it is in trauma stage (i.e. during the first few days).

○ If the receiver suffers from asthma, the prone position is normally not desirable. Do not apply deep compression to their thorax and always ask them for feedback.

○ Check whether the receiver is suffering from period pain – Thai Bodywork can really ease their condition, but it is up to the receiver whether they wish to receive on that particular day.

○ Check for skin problems such as warts, cuts and bruises, and avoid these areas.

Remember to pay attention to the Watchpoints and Benefits included throughout the book.

anatomy

Thai Bodywork is not based on the Western system of anatomy. However, most people who read this book will think of the body in these terms.

Even though experienced givers are encouraged to 'think Thai', which means to work more intuitively, they have learned the mechanics of the body they are working with, and what is likely to happen if one part of the body is pushed or stretched too far.

This means that it is necessary for everyone practising Thai Bodywork to at least be familiar with the basic muscle groups, the skeletal structure and the circulatory system.

SKELETAL STRUCTURE

❶ **Cervical vertebrae** – this upper section of the spine, the top seven vertebrae, is very flexible, allowing the head a wide range of movement. However, this flexibility makes the cervical spine particularly vulnerable to injury.

❷ **Thoracic vertebrae** – these 12 vertebrae are linked to and move with the 12 pairs of ribs. The ribs form a protective cage that shields the body's internal organs from injury.

❸ **Lumbar vertebrae** – the five vertebrae between the ribs and the pelvis bear the weight of the whole torso.

❹ **Sacral vertebrae** – these five vertebrae eventually fuse together with the coccyx to form solid bone, at about 21 years of age.

❺ **Coccyx** – the bottom four vertebrae of the spine. The tail.

❻ **Pelvis** – made up of three fused bones, this solid structure supports the lower organs and connects the upper body with the lower.

❼ **Hip joint** – ball-and-socket construction that connects the femur and pelvis.

❽ **Femur** – thigh bone.

❾ **Fibula and Tibia** – the two bones of the lower leg.

❿ **Ankle joint and Tarsals** – ankles and feet.

⓫ **Humerus** – upper arm bones.

⓬ **Radius and Ulna** – lower arm bones.

⓭ **Clavicle** – collar bone.

⓮ **Carpals, Metacarpals and Phalanges** – bones of hand and the wrist.

MUSCLE GROUPS

❶ **Biceps** (front) and **Triceps** (back) – muscles of upper arm. Used to move the arm.

❷ **Deltoid** – encloses shoulder and upper arm. Used for forward and backward movement.

❸ **Trapezius** – runs down the back of the neck and along the shoulders. Used to extend the head.

❹ **Latissimus dorsi** (lats) – runs from the mid thoracic to the lumbar region. Helps pull the shoulders down and back and the body upwards.

❺ **Rectus abdominus** (abs) – runs vertically down the entire front of the abdomen. This postural muscle draws the front of the pelvis upwards.

❻ **Gluteus maximus** – forms the buttocks. Used for running, jumping and climbing.

❼ **Semitendinosus** (one of the hamstrings) – runs down the middle of the back of the thigh. Used to extend the thigh and flex the leg at the knee.

❽ **Quadriceps extensor** – runs down the middle of the front of the thigh. It performs the opposite movement to the hamstrings.

❾ **Gastrocnemius** – forms the greater part of the calf muscles, and runs down the back of the lower leg.

ORGANS

❶ Lungs
❷ Heart (not shown)
❸ Liver
❹ Stomach
❺ Spleen (not shown)
❻ Kidneys (back)
❼ Pancreas (not shown)
❽ Small intestine
❾ Large intestine
❿ Bladder (not shown)

CIRCULATORY SYSTEM

❶ Heart
❷ Internal jugular vein
❸ Common carotid artery
❹ Superior vena cava
❺ Inferior vena cava
❻ Femoral artery (right leg)
❼ Femoral vein (left leg)
❽ Aorta

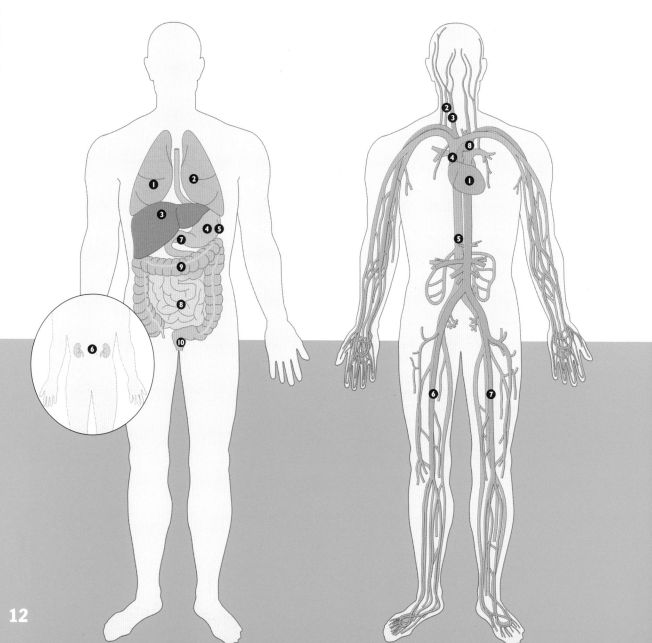

sen lines

The energy lines in Thai Bodywork are called 'Sen' lines. In theory there are 72,000 of them, but in practice far fewer are used, as shown here in the diagrams. Although they are reminiscent of the meridians used in Chinese medicine, they should not be confused with them.

While the meridians are associated with specific organs and needles, with pressure applied to certain meridians in order to increase energy flow to a particular organ, the Sen lines instead follow the form of the body and are connected to the entire body, mind and spirit.

The energy that runs through the Sen lines powers the physical, mental and emotional functions. When it is flowing smoothly and is balanced, we are free from disease. Conversely, when the energy supply is deficient or when it is blocked, we do not function so well. Thai Bodywork works on the Sen lines in two ways:

• by stretching, it helps to free the restriction to the arm by opening up surrounding interconnecting tissue.

• through applying pressure to stimulate energy flow.

The technical procedures for working on the Sen lines are described in the section on Basic Techniques (see pages 20–5).

SEN LINES (BACK)

This shows the Sen lines Itha and Pingala running up either side of the spine in what is called the laminar groove. It is important to work in the groove and not on the spine itself, as this would be both painful and dangerous to the receiver.

SEN LINES (FRONT)

① Itha – starts at the navel, runs down the front of the left thigh, turns left at the knee, ascends the back of the left thigh, ascends the left side of the spine (in laminar groove) and over the top of the head, finishing at the left nostril.

② Pingala – takes the same course as Itha, but on the right side.

③ Sumana – starts at the navel, runs straight up and inside the throat, finishing at the base of the tongue.

④ Kalatharee – starts at the navel and divides into four branches: two branches descend through the groin and down the legs, ending at the toes. The other two branches ascend to the armpits, and run down the arms, stopping at the fingers.

⑤ Sahatsarangsi – starts at the navel, descends the inner left leg, turns at the ankle and runs back up the body, through the throat and finishes at the left eye.

⑥ Tawaree – takes the same course as Sahatsarangsi, but on the right side.

⑦ Lawusang – starts at the navel, runs up through the throat and stops at the left ear.

⑧ Ulanga – takes the same course as Lawusang, but on the right side of the body.

⑨ Nantakawat – starts at the navel and divides into two branches: Sukumang – stops at the anus; Sikinee – stops at the urethra.

⑩ Kitcha – starts at the navel and descends to the sex organs: Kitchana – clitoris; Pittakun – penis.

LEG SEN LINES

Inside Leg
• Sen Line 1 starts above the ankle bone, travels along the underside of the shin bone, jumps across the knee to resurface one thumb length (receiver's) down from the centre of the patella (knee cap) and continues straight up to the crease line at groin.
• Sen Line 2 starts under the ankle bone, half-way between Sens 1 and 3, travels up the middle of the calf muscle, jumps across the knee, resurfacing two thumb lengths down from the centre of the patella and continues straight up the middle of the inner thigh to the crease line at the groin, half-way between Sen lines 1 and 3.
• Sen Line 3 starts on the inner edge of the Achilles tendon behind the ankle, travels straight up the underside of the calf muscle and jumps over the knee to resurface three thumb lengths down from the centre of the patella, ending at the start of the near-side buttock.

Outside Leg
• Sen Line 1 starts on the front side of the ankle, runs up in the groove alongside the shin bone, jumps across the knee and resurfaces one thumb length down from the centre of the patella and continues straight up to the crease line of leg/hip.
• Sen Line 2 starts above the ankle bone, runs up the centre of the calf half-way between Sens 1 and 3, jumps across the knee, resurfaces two thumb lengths down from the centre of the patella and continues up the centre of the outer thigh between Sens 1 and 3 to the crease line at the hip.
• Sen Line 3 starts under the backside of the ankle bone, sitting on the Achilles tendon, runs up along the outside edge of the calf, jumps across the knee, resurfaces three thumb lengths down from the centre of the patella and continues up the outside edge of the thigh to the crease line at the hip.

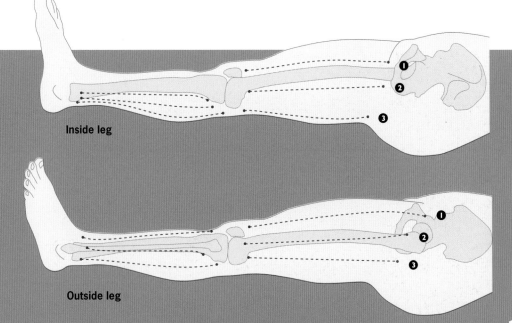

Inside leg

Outside leg

stances

When performing Thai Bodywork, the giver adopts a variety of stances. Each stance is described here, and will be referred to by name only. Descriptions of the stances are not repeated in the text, so please refer back to this section for details.

As some of these positions stretch the body and require a lot of body movement on the part of the giver, it is important to do warm-up exercises before beginning, and not to push your body into a position if you are experiencing pain.

horse

With knees wide apart, buttocks raised and your bodyweight resting on the knees while keeping the toes flexed, this stance enables the giver to work in close proximity to the receiver. The work area is aligned opposite your pelvic area (hara, see page 20). The stance can be lowered by dropping the feet or raised by lifting the body higher over the knees.

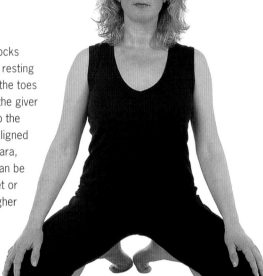

thai sitting

The giver has one leg bent beneath and pointing behind and away from the body, with the buttock resting on the heel. The other leg is bent and raised, and pointing at right angles from the first, and with the foot pointing in the same direction as the knee. This stance allows movement to travel up and down the receiver's body. It is comfortable for the giver as it supports the lower back.

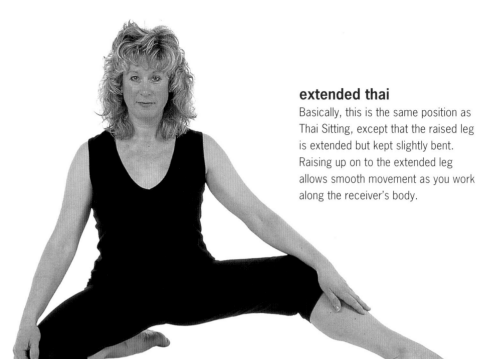

extended thai

Basically, this is the same position as Thai Sitting, except that the raised leg is extended but kept slightly bent. Raising up on to the extended leg allows smooth movement as you work along the receiver's body.

L-shaped sitting

Sitting with back straight, the giver has one leg extended and the other drawn up so the sole of the foot is placed against the opposite inner thigh. This stance is used mainly for detailed work on feet and hands. It gives support to the limb being worked on and is comfortable for the giver when they are required to work for extended periods.

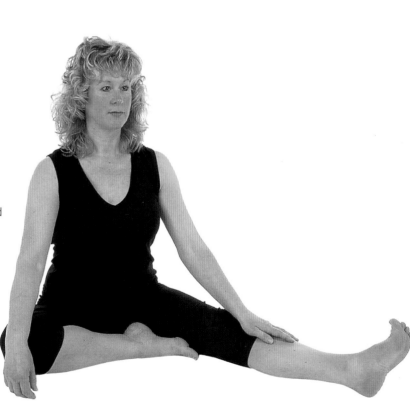

thai lunge

One leg is bent with the knee extended in front of the foot and the heel kept flat on the ground – it is this leg that supports most of the upper body weight. The back leg is extended with the knee touching the floor. The back foot may be flexed and resting on the toes or lying flat. The lunging knee's position in front of the foot allows greater body depth and closer proximity to the ground. The direction is frontal and this stance is used frequently in the supine leg section and arm stretch.

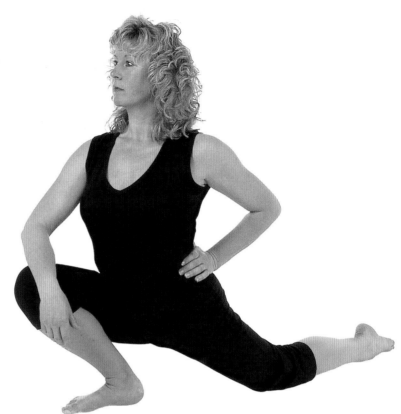

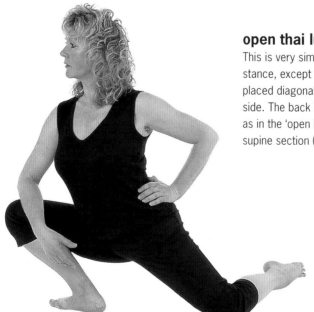

open thai lunge

This is very similar to the Thai Lunge stance, except that the front leg is placed diagonally open out towards the side. The back leg is slightly rolled in, as in the 'open leg' position in the supine section (see page 40).

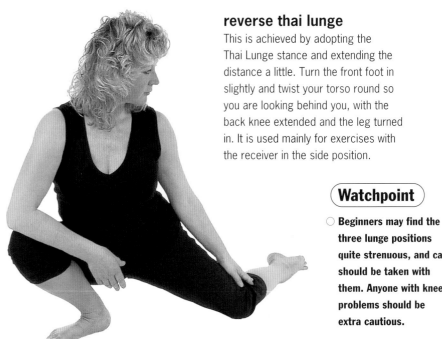

reverse thai lunge

This is achieved by adopting the Thai Lunge stance and extending the distance a little. Turn the front foot in slightly and twist your torso round so you are looking behind you, with the back knee extended and the leg turned in. It is used mainly for exercises with the receiver in the side position.

Watchpoint

○ **Beginners may find the three lunge positions quite strenuous, and care should be taken with them. Anyone with knee problems should be extra cautious.**

half kneeling

This is an upright kneeling stance, with both legs kept at right angles to the body. It is used frequently in all of the positions.

basic techniques

There are a number of techniques for working on the muscles and Sen lines, using the hands and elbows. Take some time to practise these techniques on yourself, or a friend, before beginning a full treatment. Here are a few terms you should familiarize yourself with before you start:

hello It is important to move into a new area gently so as not to shock. Hello positions facilitate this and also allow the practitioner to 'tune into' their listening skills.

listening hand A hand laid gently on the receiver. Used for sensing reaction during application.

mother hand A support hand used to give comfort or reassurance to the receiver. Its pressure is light and gentle. Can also be used as a listening hand.

hara The area which lies between the ribs and diaphragm down to the hip bones and pubic bone, the centre being the navel. This is a very powerful part of the body and is often neglected and abused. It is the seat of the emotions which often holds experiences going back to childhood. It is also known as the power centre of the body – the *tan tien*. It is the place where we direct our focus on deep breathing to relax and energize. It is also the area containing most of our internal organs including, of course, the reproductive system. It is an area that should be treated with the utmost respect and compassion.

close To relax an area (usually with palm presses) after you have applied deep pressure (usually thumb pressure) which opens the area.

points These are similar to acupressure points; that is, they are strategically placed entry points direct to the energy paths or Sen lines.

breathing Essential throughout treatment for both the practitioner and receiver. Used to help relax, to energize, for the timing of each application and to connect the physical body to the subtle body.

rock on, rock off A flowing motion of rocking bodyweight forward on to receiver and straight back off – no holding or waiting.

hook and pull When fingers bend in a curl-like position to facilitate a good hold. This is normally used for working Sen lines.

Palm Press (PP) ➤

Palm Presses (PP) are used throughout and must be used before and after you work the Sen lines to relax the limb you are working on. They prepare an area for deeper pressure work and relax the body between different procedures. There are a number of ways of using PP. The focus of contact is from the centre point of your palm 'as a warm beam of light'. Keep fingers relaxed and try not to apply pressure from the heel of your hands, as this touch is too sharp. PP is generally used in an 'alternate hand-rocking side-to-side or "penguin" motion', with the angle of delivery perpendicular to the body.

Alternate PP: Place the palms where instructed and, keeping your own body relaxed and balanced, with the arms straight, lean your weight – but not too heavily – on to one hand, then on to the other and back again, keeping up a steady rocking motion like a penguin.

To move up and down a limb, use 'hand chases hand'. As you rock on to one hand, move the other farther up the limb, rock on to it, and bring your free hand up to follow it as in open-close, open-close.

Double Palm: Rather than using the hands alternately, pressure is applied with both hands at the same time.

Hand on Hand: For this technique, place one hand over the other – with the fingers in line – and exert pressure with both hands at the same time.

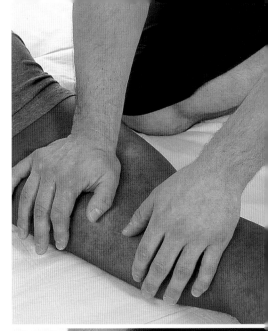

Thumb Press (TP) ➤

Thumb Presses (TP) are at the heart of working the Sen lines. Essentially TP is a similar technique to PP.

Pressure is applied by sinking the thumb pad, never from the point or the tip. To ensure this, place the thumb flat against the point you are working on. As with PP, the angle of delivery is always perpendicular. Initially avoid pressing too hard until you have developed more sensitive listening skills.

Only through observation and practice will you learn how much pressure to apply, but a rough guideline is enough to be felt but not enough to cause pain (sink the thumbs in as if sinking them into jelly). If applying pressure is deep, spiral the thumbs out clockwise.

Keep the rest of the hand relaxed or tension will flow into the thumb. Do not use TP directly on bones or on tendons.

TP is applied in the same way as PP, with either a rocking 'penguin' or 'hand chases hand' motion.

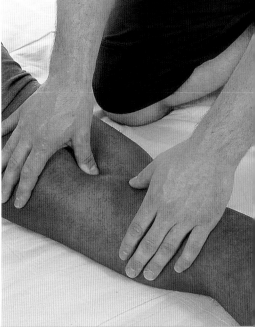

Slide Stretch ▸▸

This is a slow pulling movement used on fingers and toes.

Support the hand or foot you are working on with one hand. Grasp the finger or toe between the thumb and forefinger of the other hand, squeeze firmly and simultaneously slide the fingers along the digit. A cracking or popping sound may occur – this is nothing to worry about, nor is it the aim of the technique.

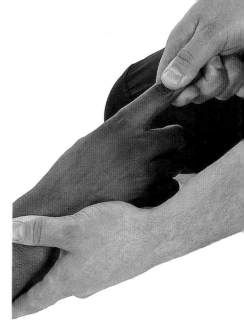

Caterpillar ▸▸

Generally applied to fingers and toes. Gently hold the digit between the thumb pad and the middle of your cupped index finger. Use alternate thumb and index finger actions, applying pressure away towards the toe or fingertip in a caterpillar-like movement.

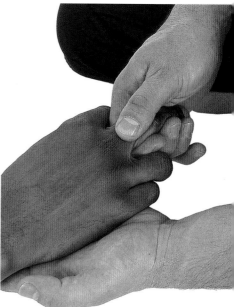

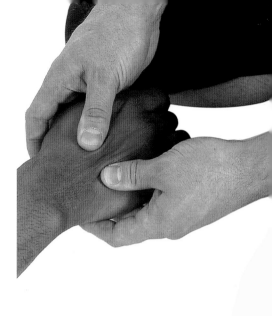

Thumb Circles (TC) ▸▸

This versatile technique can be used over all parts of the body. Using TP on bony areas such as the back of the hands or the top of the feet causes pain, which is why a more gentle circular movement of the thumbs is substituted. The giver's fingers should be relaxed yet supportive. Firmer pressure can be applied to the trapezius.

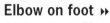

Apply pressure through the thumb pad and circle in a clockwise direction using soft to firm pressure. Always circle away from the centre of the body area. Keep your fingers relaxed.

Elbow on foot ▸▸

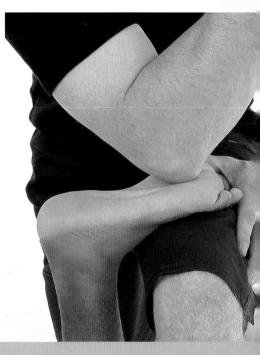

An alternative to TP, and used to apply more pressure to such areas as the sole of the foot.

Bend your arm up, keeping it relaxed. Place the point of the elbow bone to apply pressure, then release the forearm allowing the hand to drop in an opening action.

This is a powerful technique. Always apply the elbow lightly. With the arm bent and hand relaxed, gently sink the elbow into the area and release the pressure immediately by opening your arm. This technique may be applied to other areas of the body but only if the giver is at an advanced level.

Loose Fist ▸▸

Used on the back, shoulders and head to relax and revitalize.

Form loose fists and, keeping the wrists loose as well, apply alternate pummelling pressure according to the receiver's needs, making contact with your curled little fingers. Your wrists need to be relaxed as any tension in them will travel through them and be too sharp on the receiver.

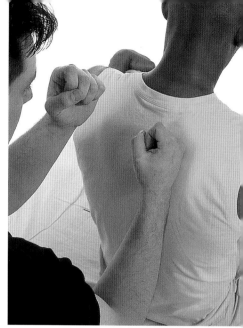

Prayerchop ▸▸

A chopping action used on the shoulders (and trapezius), back (but not over the kidneys), back of legs and shoulders.

Place hands in 'prayer' position. Open fingers, spreading hands in fan-like style. Working from loose wrists – not elbows – tap body area keeping hands together. Your elbows should be held out while working from the wrists. Pressure may be gentle to very firm. The prayerchop may also be used on the scalp.

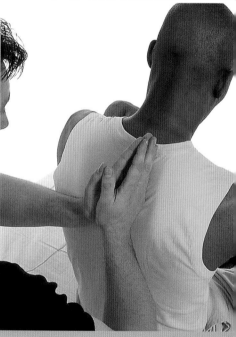

Puffer ▸▸

Similar to Loose Fist, and another versatile technique that is good for use on children and the very frail. Use for head, shoulders, back and legs.

Cup one hand and place it over the cupped palm of the other as if holding a ball, with no spaces between the fingers. Imagine you are holding a ball of light that must not be squashed. Working from the wrists, tap the body area loosely with the knuckles of the lower hand. If the technique is done correctly you will hear a puffing sound from air inside your cupped hands. Practice is generally required to achieve this very versatile and useful technique.

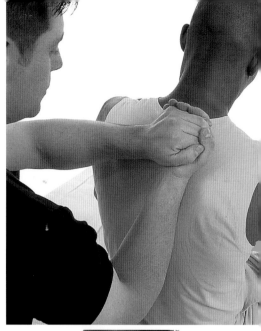

Forearm Roll ▸▸

A technique mostly used on the legs and the feet.

Keep your hand relaxed. Start with the soft underside of the arm, with your palm facing down. Roll the arm away over the area you are working on so that the palm is now turned upwards.

Take your arm off the body, smoothly turn it back over so that the palm is facing down again, move it farther along the limb, and repeat.

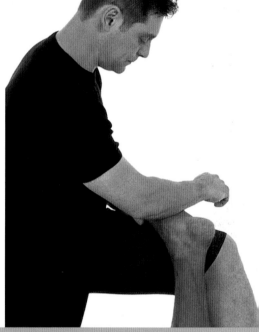

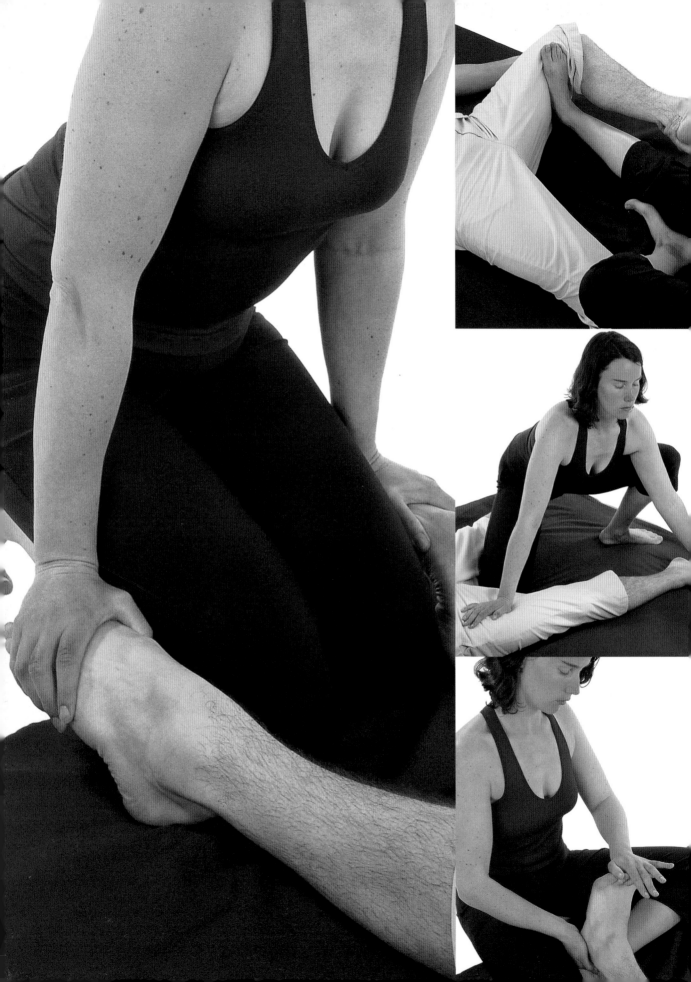

supine position

The supine position (with the receiver lying on their back) is perhaps the most frequently used in Thai Bodywork as it provides the giver with access to nearly all parts of the body. In addition, the receiver, lying on their back throughout, will find this a comfortable and relaxing position.

1 Saying Hello

Preparation
- With receiver lying on mat, kneel to their side and place a hand lightly on their hara.
- Quieten your mind, centre energy in your hara, and focus on breathing deeply in rhythm with receiver. ▸▸

2 Hello to the Feet

Watchpoints

○ **Ensure arms and back are straight when applying PP.**
○ **Check that the receiver's knees are comfortable when turning feet farther out during PP.**

Preparation
- Kneel at receiver's feet, facing them.
- Cup your hands over medial arch of each foot (see page 32).

Application
- Make alternate PP on each foot, gently rocking your body from side to side as you do it, shifting your bodyweight on to the hand applying pressure. ▸▸
- Continue to PP feet for about 30 seconds. Start with very light pressure and gradually apply firmer pressure. This will allow receiver to get used to your touch.

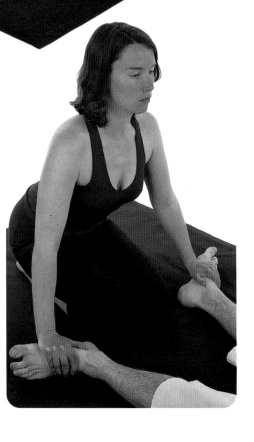

28

3 Legs

Application

- Maintaining rocking motion, PP walking up and down both legs, taking care not to press on knees. Instead, cup knees with your palms and warm them up using gentle circular movements. ⤓
- Close with alternate PP to feet.

Watchpoints

- When using PP above knee take care to avoid pressing into thigh bone.
- When giving PP ensure your weight is distributed evenly across your hand when pressing down, not concentrated in the heel of hand.

Benefits

Saying 'hello' gently to the area of body you are about to work on, especially if using TP, is vital for helping the person relax and move into a more receptive state.

29

4 Six Points of the Foot

Preparation
● Remaining between receiver's feet, (move back a little to aid angle of delivery), drape fingers slightly over medial arch (see page 32) with thumbs on soles of feet. ⤓

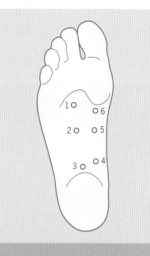

Six points of the foot
TP each point from 1–6 as shown.

Watchpoints
○ Try to keep angle of delivery perpendicular to body by turning feet out as you apply pressure.
○ Relax fingers.

Application
● Place thumbs on point 1. ▸▸
● TP point in both feet simultaneously, using your bodyweight rather than muscular force. Keep arms straight and slowly rock on/rock off.
● TP points 2, 3, 4, 5 and 6 in same way.
● Close with alternate PP of feet.

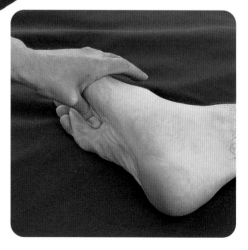

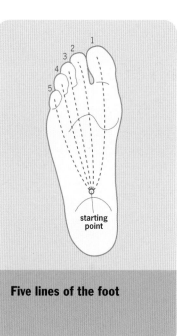

Five lines of the foot

5 Five Lines of the Foot

Application

- Working both feet at same time, and with thumbs on soles, begin with TP in a straight line from starting point to big toe. ▸▸
- At ball of the foot, do not press into bone, but use TC. Continue to TC up to big toe.
- At big toe, lightly squeeze tip of toe.
- Repeat with TP and TC from starting point to each toe in turn.
- Close with alternate PP of feet.

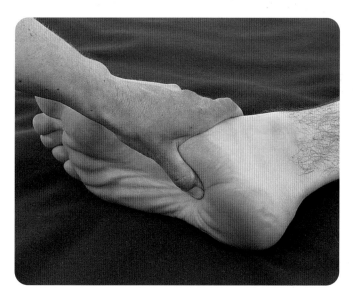

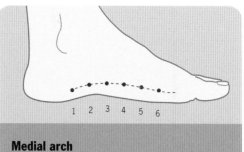

Medial arch
Use TP on points following arch/instep of the foot.

6 Medial Arch

Application

● Working both feet at same time, and starting at point 1, TP along points towards ball of foot and back again. Rock on/rock off very slowly. ▶▶

● Close with alternate PP of feet.

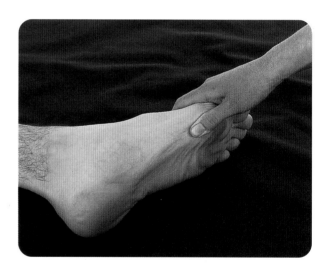

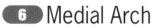

Watchpoints

○ Pay attention to receiver's response when working on top of feet. This is a sensitive area for many people, so work slowly and carefully.

○ Apply very light TP on pregnant women.

Benefit
Great for tired feet.

7 # Four Lines of
the Foot

Preparation
● Place feet in upright position and
support them with your fingers. ⌄

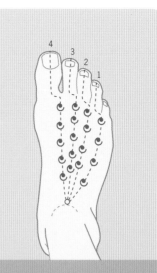

Four lines of the foot
**Starting point is in hollow at centre
front of ankle.**

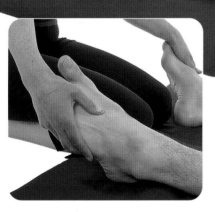

Application
● Beginning at starting point, TC
down groove between first and
second toes (easy to find as it is
defined by large tendons). ◀◀

(**Watchpoint**)

○ **Never TP on bone, only
on soft tissue. Use TC
or Caterpillar on toes
and fingers.**

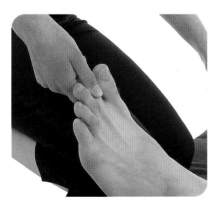

● Caterpillar along toes and
slide off. ◀◀
● Repeat along remaining lines.
● Close with alternate PP of feet.

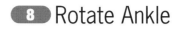

8 Rotate Ankle

Preparation

- Maintaining contact with receiver by holding their foot, bring yourself into L-shaped Sitting position.
- Hold foot with heel resting in palm of hand. Cup toes with other hand. ⥥

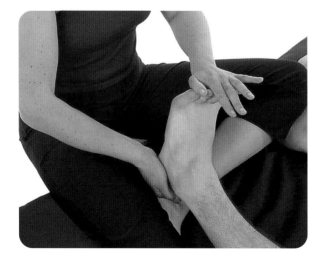

Application

- Keeping heel steady, slowly rotate ankle fully in one direction three times, and then three times in reverse direction. Receiver should feel sensation all the way up to their neck. ◄◄

9 Twist Foot

Application

- Keeping heel steady with inside hand, use other hand to grasp foot across medial arch (see page 32), starting at heel end. ▸▸
- Leaning back, draw elbows in, applying equal force to both hands, to help twist foot gently outwards.
- Repeat move two or three times towards big toe and back again.

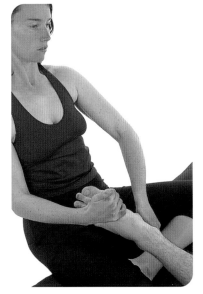

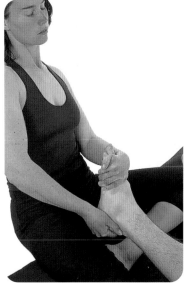

- Change hands and repeat on other side of foot, twisting it in this time. ▸▸

10 Stretch Toes

Application

- Move back a little and place receiver's foot on floor.
- Take big toe at joint nearest foot between thumb and index finger, placing your 'mother' hand (see page 20) over the top for support.
- Rotate it two or three times in each direction to loosen joint. Breathe in, then firmly pull toe towards you on out breath. Sometimes toe may 'crack', but this is not the aim.
- Repeat on each toe. ▸▸
- Finish by stroking foot gently to relax it.
- **Repeat movements 8, 9 and 10 on other foot.**

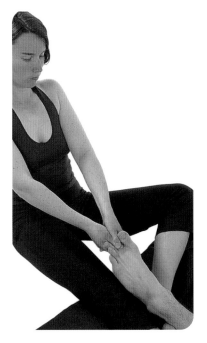

Watchpoints

- ○ **Work with a straight back. Application comes from hara not from your arms.**
- ○ **Do not bend forwards with head dropped.**
- ○ **Apply on out breath.**

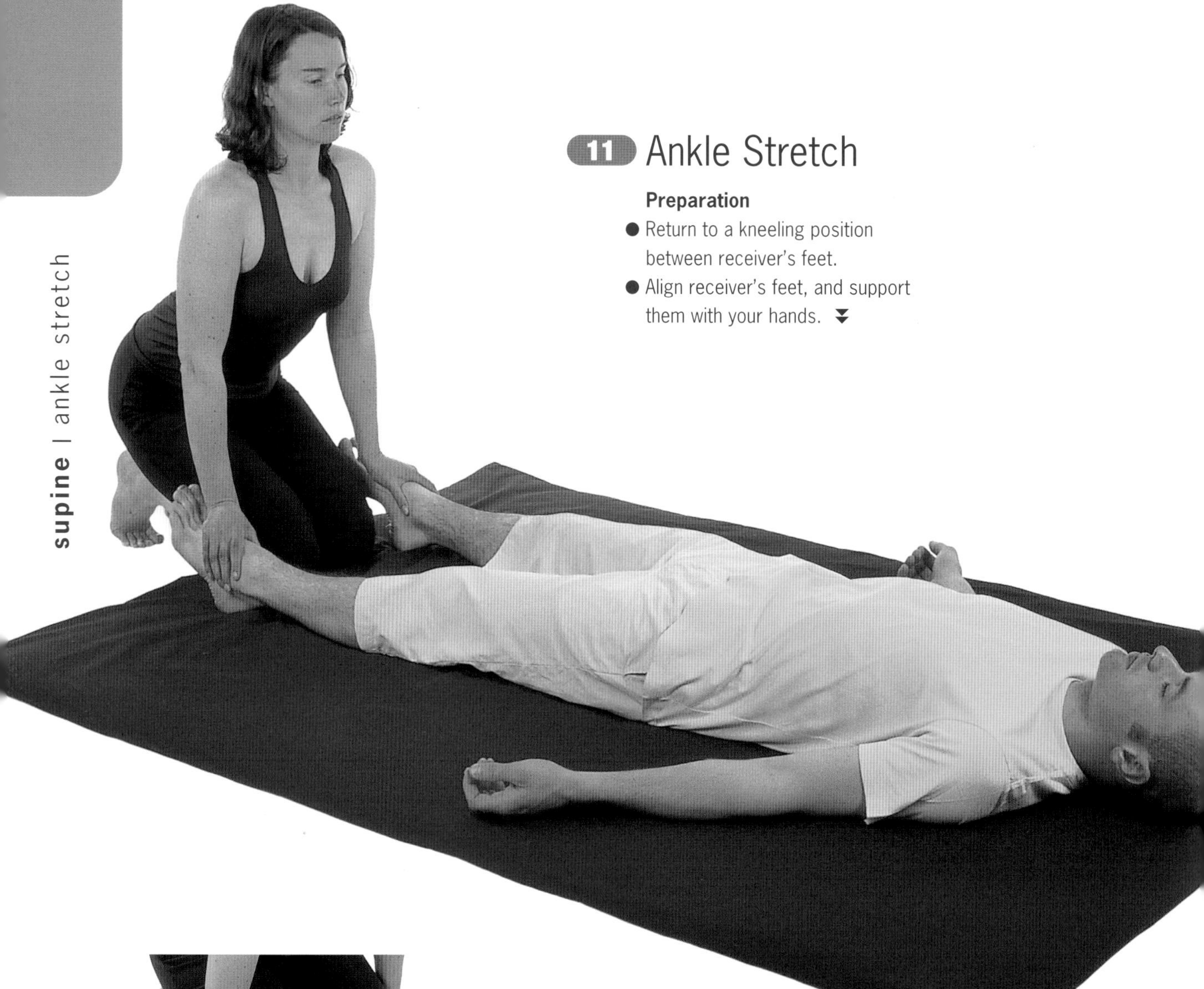

11 Ankle Stretch

Preparation

- Return to a kneeling position between receiver's feet.
- Align receiver's feet, and support them with your hands.

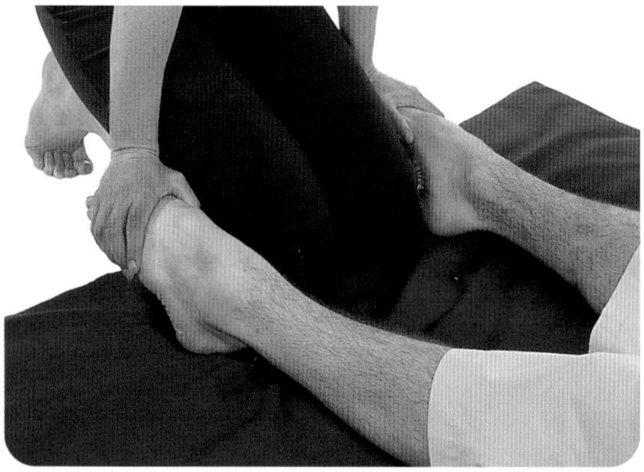

Application

- Use double palm compression slowly from ankle to toes in a 1-2-3-2-1 sequence. Keep pressure softer at ankle and increase it as you move to toes.

12 Ankle Flex

Application

● Move well back from receiver, and working both feet together, cup receiver's toes.

● Push toes forwards by leaning in, then release. Repeat three times. ▸▸

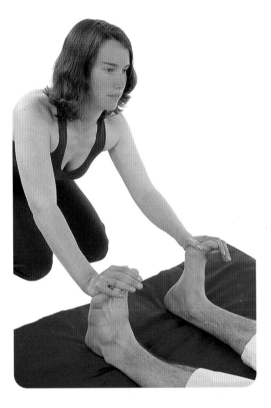

13 Cross Feet

Application

● Place one foot to lie across other.

● Place one hand to hold feet in position and with other hand PP in a 1-2-3-2-1 sequence starting at ankle and working towards toes of top foot. ▸▸

● Reverse feet, and repeat.

● Close with alternate PP of feet.

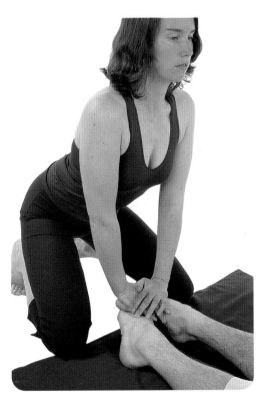

Benefits
Loosens ankle joint and Achilles tendon.

14 Outside Leg

Preparation

- To work Sen lines adopt a wide Horse stance, with pelvis opposite receiver's knee.
- Start by turning foot in with one hand on outside edge of foot and other at hip bone, fingers pointing outwards.
- Breathe in and on out breath rock on and off, using your bodyweight to stretch the leg.
- Using both hands, PP in to knee, PP out, PP in and PP down to ankle.
- Place your foot against receiver's to prevent it rolling out as you work on it during application. ⯮

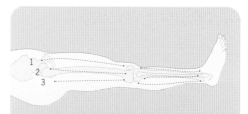

Outside leg

Follow line 1 deep in the groove on near side of the shin bone until it curves down just before knee. Then measure one thumb length from centre of top of patella (knee cap) towards you and continue up the thigh.

To measure Sen line 2 at knee, use two thumb lengths, and three for Sen line 3.

Watchpoints

- ○ Do not apply any TP to lower leg if receiver is pregnant, only PP.
- ○ Points directly above knee are tender – travel lightly!

Application

- Following Line 1 on diagram, TP from the ankle to hip and return. ▸▸
- Repeat for Lines 2 and 3.
- Close with PP up leg and back to ankle.

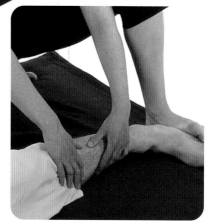

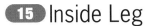 ## 15 Inside Leg

Preparation

- To work Sen lines, open receiver's legs a little wider and place yourself between them in Thai sitting stance. (If you are tall and the receiver is short, you may adopt an open Thai lunge position that straddles legs.)
- Place one hand on inside edge of receiver's foot near ankle, and other towards hip bone. Using your bodyweight, rock on/rock off, gently stretching entire leg from pelvis to ankle. ▸▸
- Using both hands, PP in, PP out, PP in and PP down to ankle.

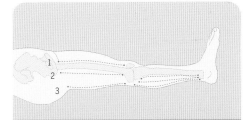

Inside leg

Note that all three inside leg lines begin in the hollow between ankle bone and Achilles tendon.

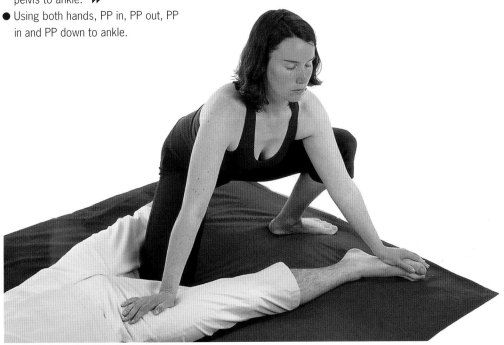

Application

- Starting at ankle, use alternate TP up line 1 and back to ankle. ▸▸
- Repeat on lines 2 and 3.
- Close with PP up leg and back to ankle.
- **Move to other side of receiver and repeat 14 and 15**.
- At completion of all Sen lines, (approximately 15 minutes) move to base of feet and integrate both legs by applying PP up and down both legs to close.

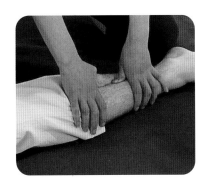

Watchpoints

- ○ Keep your back straight at all times. Rounding your back or dropping your head will result in back strain.
- ○ Remember to breathe!
- ○ Do not adjust position while applying pressure.
- ○ Remember to use a rocking motion on both PP and TP.

16 Open Leg

Preparation

- Bend receiver's leg out and place their foot against calf of other, extended leg.
- Position yourself so that you are in line with thigh of bent leg.
- If receiver's leg is high off the ground when bent, support it with a cushion.

Application

- Begin gently with hands at knee. PP with one hand to ankle and the other on thigh, working hands simultaneously and returning both back to knee.
- With fingers pointing outwards do simultaneous PP from knee to hip and back again in a 1-2-3-2-1 sequence. Slowly increase pressure as you go up, so that it is very gentle at knee and strongest at hip. ⌄
- PP in walking style down to foot again.

Watchpoint

○ This is the first time you open the groin and hip flexors, so be very gentle initially, and work towards getting firmer.

17 Open Groin

Preparation
- Sit between receiver's legs, and drape your inside leg over receiver's extended leg. Slide your outer hand to support receiver's foot on bent leg from underneath.
- Place sole of your foot (outside leg) on receiver's thigh near knee. ▶▶

Application
- Using instep, apply foot compression along inside thigh, travelling towards groin and back, allowing leg freedom to stretch open on application.

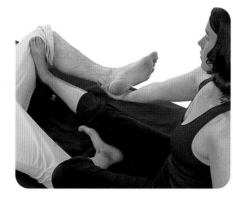

Watchpoints
- During delivery, knee of bent leg should not drop lower than hip level – it should be at a right angle or higher than hip.
- Ensure receiver's bent leg is relaxed. If it is not, ask them to breathe out and let go so that leg's weight is controlled by you, not by them.
- Angle your foot to respect the area around the groin.

18 Lock Leg

Application
- Drape receiver's bent leg over your outside leg and support by holding their heel for resistance.
- Apply foot compression along inside thigh keeping heel as low to ground as possible, travelling towards groin and back. ▶▶

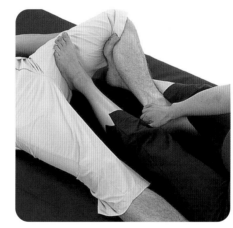

Watchpoint
- As your foot travels close to receiver's groin, angle your foot at that point for their comfort.

19 Feet Walk

Application
- Release receiver's leg and support foot as in 17. Use alternate foot compression along inner thigh to groin and back. ▶▶

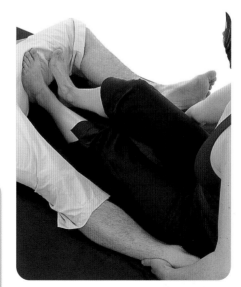

Benefits
17, 18 and 19 are popular techniques for powerfully, yet safely, opening groin, hip flexors and inside thigh.

20 Hook and Pull

Preparation
- Move to kneeling position.
- Make sure receiver's foot is as close as possible to buttocks.
- Place receiver's leg between your knees to stabilize it.
- Cross hands and place fingertips along outside 1 and inside 1 Sen lines (see page 15).

Application
- Hook and pull towards centre Sen line in a twisting movement, across thigh muscles, one hand following other, travelling to hip and back to knee. ◀◀

21 Hip Flexor Stretch

Application
- In same position, interlace your fingers and place them over top of thigh.
- Lean your body back to pull on leg, lifting hip increasingly off floor, and stretching front thigh three times, travelling to hip and back. ▶▶

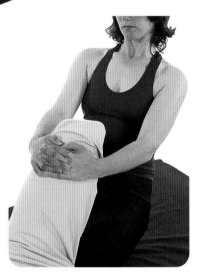

22 Ice Pick

Application
- Still with fingers interlaced, place thumbs on the inner and outer Sen lines 1. Apply TP up thigh and back again in a 'closing action' by lowering elbows a little on application. ▶▶

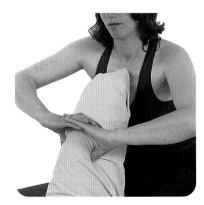

Benefits
20 and 22 are good for energy lines in front thigh. 21 opens up hip flexor and lower back.

42

23 Hamstring Compression

Application

- Moving receiver's foot forward slightly so that leg is opened up, place your thumbs together on centre Sen line on the back of thigh.
- Using simultaneous TP, work up thigh, applying firm pressure to this area. ▶▶

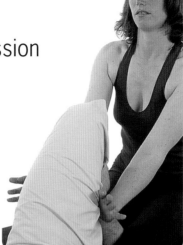

Watchpoint

○ **Keep arms straight during TP.**

24 Open Calf

Application

- Hook your fingertips into centre Sen line on back of calf at knee.
- Lean back and slowly pull in then outwards with both hands simultaneously, three or four times, travelling down line. ▶▶
- Walk back up line using alternate hands.

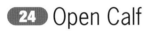

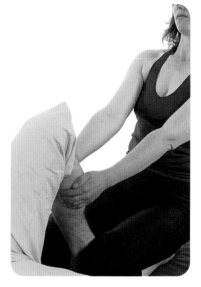

25 Nutcracker

Application

- Interlacing your fingers, clasp calf muscle with your palms.
- Press sides of calf muscle firmly with heels of your hands and push muscle away from you. Work from knee down to lower calf and back up. ▶▶
- Close by shaking calf gently with thumb and index finger.

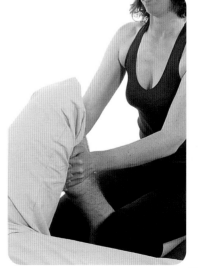

Benefits

23 is great for releasing and relaxing hamstring muscles. 24 and 25 release tension in calf muscles. Receiver may laugh as a release of ticklishness.

26 Knee to Chest

Preparation

- Move into Half Kneeling position. Bend receiver's leg, placing their foot in the crease of your thigh and groin. The foot of your bent leg should be alongside receiver's waist.
- Support bent leg by holding it at knee, and place your other hand on receiver's extended leg at top of thigh, as a listening hand, not for compression.
- If receiver is 'holding', ask them to breathe and let go.

Application

- Slowly move into a lunge, pressing against receiver's foot. This will stretch the leg. Be careful not to push too far. ⤓
- While lunging, move your inner hand in a 1-2-3-2-1 sequence from hip to knee and back. (Hand moves each time you lunge.)
- Aim receiver's knee towards their same-side shoulder.

27 Butterfly

Watchpoint

○ **If receiver has a long abdomen, large rib cage, constipation or is pregnant, direct lunge leg more towards armpit.**

Benefits

A powerful stretch for hamstrings, buttocks and opposite front thigh. Aids opening of pelvic area. Good for lower back.

Application

- In the same position, place both hands on the back of the thigh with fingers pointing outwards.
- Extend your lunge, at the same time pressing down on the thigh with straight arms in a double palm compression. This will increase the extension. ▸▸
- Continue from the knee to the pelvic bone and back in a 1-2-3-2-1 sequence.

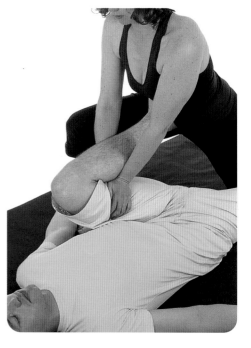

28 Open Leg Curl

Preparation

● Open your lunge to a diagonally oblique angle.
● Still support receiver's bent knee with one hand and allow receiver's leg to fall open.

Application

● Gently lower lunge stance outwards and at the same time PP receiver's upper inner thigh. ⌄

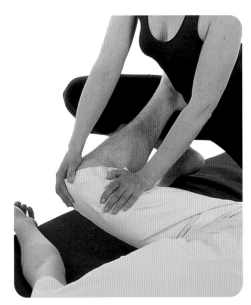

● Move angle of delivery to a forward one by rotating your outer hip forwards, simultaneously pushing receiver's leg in direction of their armpit, creating a curl. ◄◄
● Repeat whole action with compression hand travelling in a 1-2-3-2-1 sequence from groin to knee.

Benefits

This powerful stretch opens hip flexor, stretches inner and back thigh, and with compressions stimulates Sen lines.

45

29 Hamstring Stretch

Preparation

● Move back into Half Kneeling position, hold receiver's ankle with your hand and raise leg towards their torso in direction of opposite shoulder, allowing leg to be bent but not floppy.

Application

● With other hand just above back of the knee, gently compress on thigh. Simutaneously lunging forward and back, repeat PP to buttock and back of leg in a 1-2-3-2-1 sequence. ▸▸

● As you press thigh and lunge, gently push receiver's foot forwards, extending stretch.

Watchpoint

○ Be careful. This is a strong stretch. Do not try to straighten receiver's leg. Be sensitive and ask for feedback during delivery.

30 Ninety Degrees

Preparation

● Move to a sitting position, and ensure you are close enough for your feet to reach receiver's outside hip.

● Support heel with your outside hand, and with other hand hold above arch of foot.

● With receiver's knee at a right angle to thigh, place your outside foot on thigh just above back of knee, with sole placed crosswise.

Application

● Push against thigh, straightening your leg and pulling receiver's heel towards you as you do. ⌄

● Repeat foot compression along the back of thigh in a 1-2-1 sequence. On second compression be gentle, keeping receiver's leg at a right angle at all times.

Benefits

Opens knee joint.
Stretches Achilles tendon.

31 Bent Out

Preparation

- Gently bend receiver's leg out and back so their foot is pointing towards their head. Check receiver is comfortable.
- Position yourself at receiver's knee in Horse stance, as you prepare to work on opening hip and thigh. If receiver is not flexible, support knee with a cushion or rest it on your closed thighs.

Application

- PP thigh with both hands simultaneously in butterfly position from knee to hip, starting very gently and getting firmer. ▶▶

- Slide one hand along to knee and gently, with both hands, compress and stretch upper thigh. ▶▶
- Prayerchop down and up thigh finishing at knee. Then stroke down.
- Finish by slowly straightening out leg, laying it next to other, and rubbing knee in a circular motion.

Benefits

Opens hip flexor and front thigh. Opens energy lines in the lower abdominal muscles.

47

32 Calf Stretch

Preparation
- In Half Kneeling position move to outside of leg.
- Hold receiver's heel in one palm, with their foot along your forearm. Place your other hand on their thigh as listening hand only.

Application
- Flex their foot by leaning away and pulling your elbow down, stretching lower calf and Achilles tendon. Repeat three times. ⤵
- Release leg by lunging receiver's knee gently to their shoulder.

33 Cross Twist

Application

- Still in Half Kneeling position, move your body round to face receiver, very slowly bringing their leg across their body so thigh lies at a right angle to torso.
- Place one hand on upper knee and other on shoulder. Ask receiver to breathe in, and on out breath tell receiver to relax.
- Allow leg to lower itself as lower back opens up. ▶▶
- On each out breath receiver relaxes leg a little more, allowing it to fall closer to floor.
- **Repeat from 16 to 33 on other side.**

Watchpoints

- Must be applied very slowly with feedback.
- Do not lean on receiver or use compression. Instead, help them to keep shoulders on the floor, using the out breath to relax them. This will help diagonal cross twist.
- Help leg return very slowly, so that lower lumbar area returns gently to normal.
- Do not do this if receiver has recently slipped a disc or has had recent abdominal surgery.

Benefits

Releases lower back, mid-lumbar and thoracic spine. Opens pectorals and chest. Stretches outer thigh into buttock. Connects and opens various energy lines. Helps release large intestine.

49

34 Half Plough

Preparation

- Lift both receiver's legs to right angles to floor.
- Standing behind receiver's buttocks, cup both their heels in inner-side hand, and support with other hand.
- Move into Lunge position with front leg in line with receiver's waist level.
- Ask receiver to place their hands on their knees. Tell them that during delivery they will feel some resistance but to keep their arms straight throughout movement. ⌄

Watchpoints

- ○ Take care to deliver action to both legs equally.
- ○ Keep legs equally balanced or hips will swing to one side.
- ○ Keep your shoulders square to front.
- ○ Not to be used if receiver has high blood pressure.

Application

- Ask receiver to breath in. On out breath extend your lunge and push both feet forwards together until feet are over the receiver's face. Hold for a few seconds and return very slowly. ▸▸

Benefits

Good for lower back, digestion and heart. Redirects blocked energy in legs, shoulders and neck.

35 Buttock Stretch

Preparation
● Adopt Thai Half Kneeling stance. Place one of receiver's legs on your shoulder. Hold other leg by ankle and cross it over first leg. Receiver's knee should be in the centre of their chest.

Application
● With your free hand, PP back of bent leg from knee to buttocks in a 1-2-3-2-1 sequence. ▶▶
● Each time you compress, rock your body forward.
● **Repeat on other side.**

Benefits
Powerful buttock and back of thigh stretcher.

36 Step In and Out

Preparation

● Holding receiver's ankles, ask them to relax. Step one foot through to rest at the side of their body at waist level. Follow with second leg, allowing their feet to rest behind you, as shown. ◀◀

Watchpoints

○ **Breathing is important.**
○ **Ease gently into Frog. If feet don't come together easily, don't force them.**
○ **Be careful not to crush ribcage with your lower legs.**
○ **Do not use if person has high blood pressure, hiatus hernia, acute asthma or a recent spinal injury.**

Benefits

Excellent for opening spine from base to neck.

37 Frog

Application

● Ask receiver to breathe in, and on out breath slowly and gradually bring their legs in front of you. Bring the soles of feet together, if possible; if not leave them open.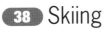

38 Skiing

Application

● Ask receiver to take a deep breath, and on out breath, bend your knees and extend your arms, pushing receiver's feet forwards. ▸▸
● Then pull back and up.
● **Repeat three times.**
● Allow legs to fall behind you, as in preparation, and carefully step out, one leg at a time.
● Lay receiver's legs on the floor.

39 Hello to the Hara

Preparation

- Before beginning work on Hara (see page 20), make sure receiver is lying comfortably. Work on this area should not be done within two hours of receiver eating.
- Kneeling beside receiver, place one palm on hara (over navel). Do not apply weight.
- Gently hold hand there and breathe in unison with receiver. ▸▸
- Ask receiver to breathe into your hand.
- Allow time for breathing. Sometimes up to 20 deep, slow breaths are required for a receiver who is used to shallow breathing.

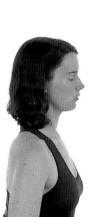

Watchpoints

- Always breathe in through the nose.
- If receiver has difficulty with slow/long in or out breaths apply rhythm breathing, starting with in for three slow counts, and out for three, increasing gradually to six.
- It is important to be patient, until receiver draws energy 'breath' down to lower abdominals.

40 Warm Up – Circling

Preparation
- Sit in Horse stance as close to receiver as possible.

Application
- With one hand placed over the other, very gently circle hara in a clockwise direction. ⩣
- This technique is used in between other techniques to integrate.
- Upper hand is used as mother hand only.

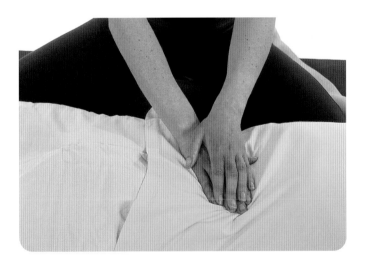

Benefits
39 and 40 help to deepen breathing, aid relaxation and relax the organs in that area: diaphragm, stomach, liver, large and small intestines.
Helps to relieve irritable bowel syndrome, middle and lower back pain, diverticulitis and period pains.

Push

Application

● Gently, but firmly, push heels of both hands in direction of navel on out breath. ▸▸

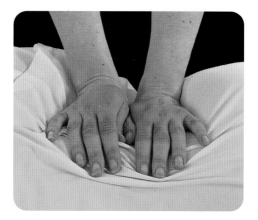

42 Pull

Application

● Angle your hands so fingers are pointing downwards (but not perpendicular), then draw them towards navel. Cup your hands over navel and bring them back to 'Push' position. ▸▸

● Repeat 'Push' and 'Pull' several times until hara area feels soft and relaxed.

● You may travel lower towards hips and then higher towards ribs.

● Finish with circling palms as in 40.

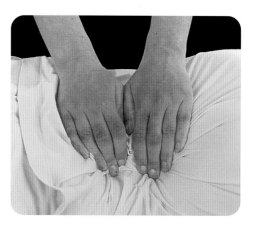

Benefits

The benefits are similar to 39 and 40, but here work goes much deeper, touching the emotional body. Receivers may experience an emotional release such as crying or laughing, or simply feel an enormous sense of freedom in this area.
Can help sciatica and lower back pain, and is good for menstrual pain or associated problems.

Watchpoints

○ **Depending on size of individual's hara and size of your hands, travelling may be limited.**

○ **This technique may be tender to blocked areas – continue gently as it helps to 'release'.**

○ **Do not do this if receiver has had surgery in last three months.**

○ **Do not apply 40–42 to pregnant women.**

43 Six Points

Preparation

- Adopt a respectful straddle position over receiver.
- Make sure you are high enough over waist so that you can work on the points vertically. Align your shoulders to make a straight line down to thumb.

Six points

The distance between points is relative to size of the hara. However, a rough guide is that each point is about a thumb's length from the navel.

Watchpoint

○ **Guiding receiver's breathing is essential as this technique can be painful if a lot of emotions are held. If it is painful, spiral your thumbs out of the points.**

Application

- It is most important to guide receiver's breathing so it is in unison with yours. Ask receiver to inhale, and on out breath sink your thumbs into each point. Pull out on an in breath, and sink in again on an out breath. ▸▸
- Using both hands simultaneously, TP points as follows:
  1 and 2 together
  3a and 4a together
  3 and 4 together
  5 and 6 together
  3 and 4 together.
- Return to side of receiver.
- **Repeat 40 again.**
- Place one hand on receiver and close this sequence with receiver deep breathing for at least eight breaths, drawing the energy down to hara.

44 Chest

Preparation
● Move to a Half Kneeling stance over receiver, at waist level.

Application
● Placing hand on hand, and using your middle fingers, do finger circles up whole length of sternum. ▸▸
● Opening hands, move to clavicle and finger circle from the centre out and back along its lower edge, using both hands simultaneously.

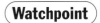

45 Ribs

Application
● Now work spaces between ribs (intercostals) in same way, moving from inside to outside then lowering to next rib space. ▸▸
● Return back up via sternum.

(**Watchpoint**)

○ **When working on a woman, exclude the breast area.**

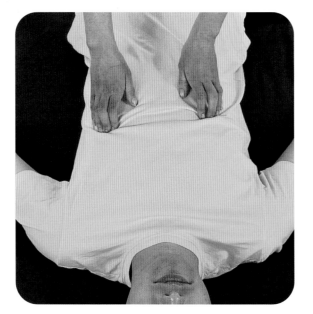

Benefits
Receiver may 'release' in both physical and emotional ways. Reactions can include laughing or tearfulness. Heightened senses can bring powerful relaxation. Good for lungs.

46 Shoulders

Application

● Moving farther up over receiver, place heels of your hands on outer edge of shoulders. Position hands so they are cupping shoulders.

● Keeping arms straight, ask receiver to breathe in, and on out breath lean in slowly but firmly for a double palm compression. Release after 2–4 seconds. ▶▶

47 Trapezius

Application

● Staying in same position, hook your fingers over the back of shoulders.

● Pull back, and lift shoulders slightly off floor. Receiver's head and chin will tilt back slightly. ▶▶

● Release slowly and ask receiver to drop their chin down, so as to align back of neck.

● Massage shoulder (trapezius) muscles well.

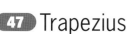

Watchpoint

○ **Make sure you are directly over receiver so angle of delivery is perpendicular to body and not diagonal.**

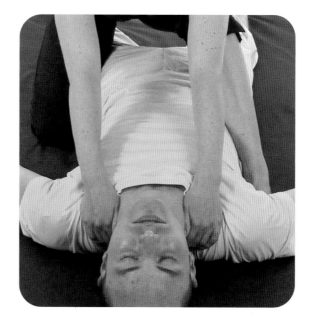

59

Watchpoints

○ Be careful not to PP directly on to joints, i.e. elbows, wrists or fingers.

○ Keep a straight back on delivery.

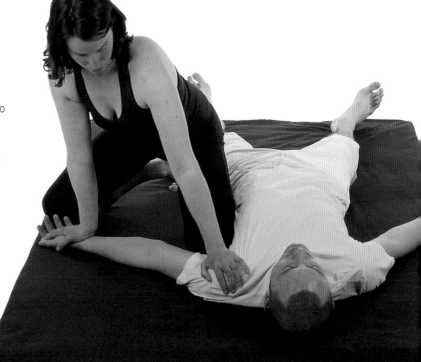

Inside arm sen line

48 Inside Arm

Preparation

● In Horse stance, kneel beside receiver and extend their arm out to side, with palm up.

● Place one hand on their wrist, the other on their shoulder, fingers pointing outwards.

Application

● Breathe in and gently compress down for 'hello' stretch. ▸▸

● Apply alternate PP in to elbow, PP out, PP in, then PP down to hand.

49 Inside Sen Line

Application

● Using both thumbs, apply alternate TP up centre line from wrist to elbow using rocking side-to-side motion. Firm pressure may be applied. Continue above elbow, between muscle and bone using lighter pressure to shoulder. ▸▸

● Work back down with TP following same line.

● PP from wrist to shoulder.

● Finish with hand on hand compression to hand.

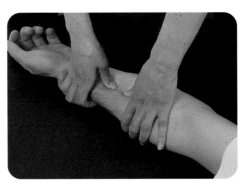

Benefit

Working on arms allows energy originating in chest area to be released even more.

Watchpoint

○ People's elbow joints differ, and with some the upper arm may not roll over to allow you to PP with ease.

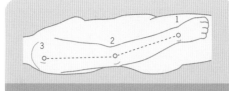

Outside arm sen line

50 Outside Arm

Preparation

- Move round to side of receiver so you are facing side of their body.
- Bring receiver's arm closer to body.
- Adopt raised Horse stance.
- Place one hand on wrist and other on shoulder and gently compress for 'hello' stretch. ▸▸

Application

- As with working inside arm, PP in to elbow, PP out, PP in, PP down to hand.

51 Outside Sen Line

Application

- TP outside centre line of arm from wrist to elbow (see diagram). ▸▸
- Continue from elbow up to shoulder, again working between muscle and the bone. Return TP to wrist.
- PP up and PP down arm.
- Finish with hand on hand compression to hand.

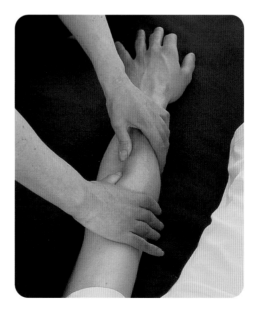

Watchpoint

○ Ask the receiver if they
have arthritis. If they
do, you may still give
treatment, but with very
light pressure.

52 Break Bread

Preparation
● Kneeling beside receiver, take their
hand and rest it on your knee.
● Support hand by lacing your own
fingers underneath receiver's first,
third and fourth fingers (or simply
interlace your fingers). This leaves
your thumbs free to work points.

Application
● Work the hand as if breaking bread
– apply pressure on the points and
turn outwards (photograph shows
hand when application is repeated
on other side). ▶▶

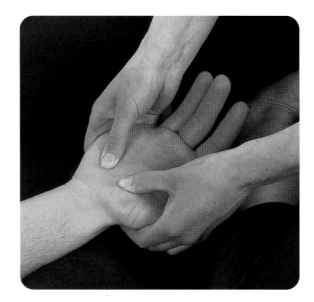

53 Six Points of
the Palm

Application
● Starting at the heel of the hand,
TP points 1 and 2 together. Then TP
3 and 4, finally 5 and 6. Use firm
pressure.
● TP palm of hand at random.
● Finish by 'breaking bread' again.

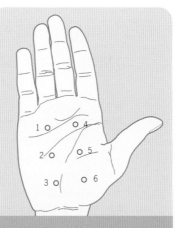

Six points of the palm
The six points are arranged around the
palm area from just below the fingers
to the heel of the hand.

Benefits
Stimulates Sen lines, releases tension and is very soothing and relaxing.

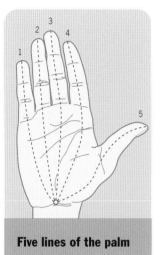

Five lines of the palm

54 ▶ Five Lines of the Palm

Preparation
● Hold hand loosely in your own hands, with your fingers free to work palm.

Application
● Beginning at centre of heel of hand, TP along the lines to base of each finger. When you reach carpal bone, change to Caterpillar technique, and circle along bone and out to end of the finger, and off. ▶▶
● You can work one line at a time, or – as shown – use both hands to work two lines simultaneously.
● Finish with 'breaking bread'.

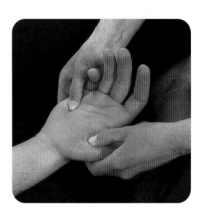

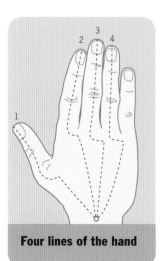

Four lines of the hand

55 ▶ Four Lines of the Hand

Application
● Turn receiver's hand over.
● Using Thumb Circles (TC), work from the starting point at centre of wrist joint. Be sure to follow lines between tendons, i.e. the grooves between fingers. ▶▶
● At knuckles, apply Caterpillar technique to end of finger and slide off. For little finger, TC up outside of hand, and off.

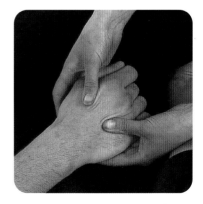

56 Rotate Wrist

Preparation
● Hold receiver's wrist gently with one hand, and lace your fingers through theirs with the other. ▶▶

Application
● Rotate receiver's wrist three times in each direction.
● Then slide your fingers out.

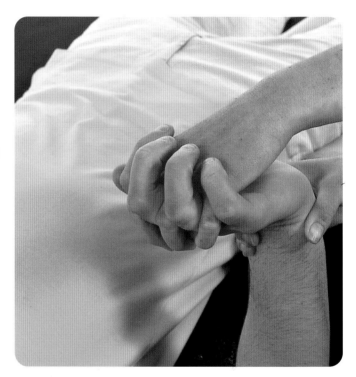

Benefits
56, 57 and 58 help to release build-ups and blockages in the hands. Done very gently, will benefit even arthritic hands.

57 Release and Stretch Fingers

Preparation
- Still supporting receiver's wrist, take each finger in turn, hold them between your second and third fingers, as shown.

Application
- Rotate finger in both directions loosely, and finally grip and slowly, Slide Stretch finger. It may 'pop', but that is alright. However, focus on stretching fingers rather than pulling them. ▸▸

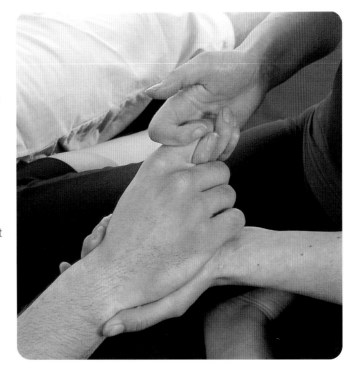

58 Caterpillar Stretch

Application
- Starting in centre of palm, knead and push fingers back using your thumbs in Caterpillar style. ▸▸
- Start with thumb and little finger simultaneously and walk in to next two fingers, as shown, followed by centre finger.

(Watchpoint)
- ○ **Do not stretch fingers back too far, and support backs of receivers' fingers with your own.**

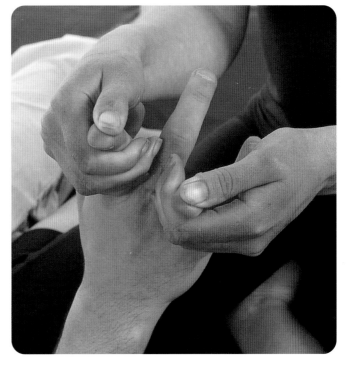

59 Side Stretch

Preparation
● Move well up receiver's body into a Thai Lunge stance to shoulder level.

Application
● Move receiver's arm gently over their head, holding it at wrist.
● Ask receiver to breathe in, and on out breath stretch their arm directly ahead of you. ▸▸

● Supporting arm, move around their head. Bringing other arm around, lean back and pull simultaneously to stretch on out breath. ▸▸
● **Repeat on other arm from 48.**

60 Neck Stretch

Preparation
- Sitting behind receiver's head, place your hands on their shoulders with your fingers pointing down their back.
- Gently knead trapezius. ▸▸
- Place receiver's head in your hands, raising it slightly off floor.

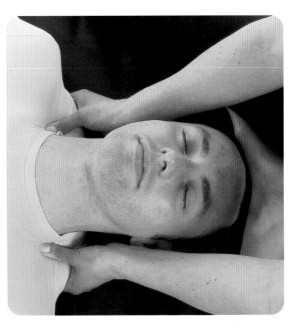

Application
- With your hands at base of skull, fingers cupping occipital bone, ask receiver to breathe in. On out breath, slowly but firmly pull head towards you. ▸▸
- **Release and repeat.**

Watchpoint
○ **If receiver has curvature on back of neck, preventing chin relaxing in alignment with body, lift head higher off floor before delivery.**

Benefits
59 opens up intercostals and armpit, abdominals and chest. Stimulates lungs.
60 opens cervical part of spine and releases tension in neck and trapezius.

61 Neck Massage

Preparation
- Place head in right hand and turn it to right.

Application
- TC along neck, then TP, pushing thumb away from spine. ▸▸
- Indulge this area, turn head gently to the other side and repeat.

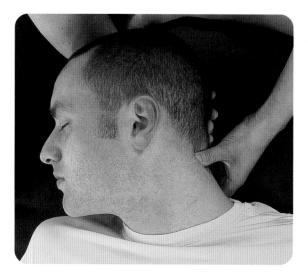

62 Neck Side Stretch

Preparation
- Place receiver's head on mat.
- Gently turn the head to the right. Place your right hand so that it is cupping side of head, including ear. Do not pull this hand – use it only as support.

Application
- Ask receiver to breathe in. With other hand cup the shoulder. On out breath, slowly stretch shoulder away from head. ▸▸
- Release and slowly turn head to other side and repeat.

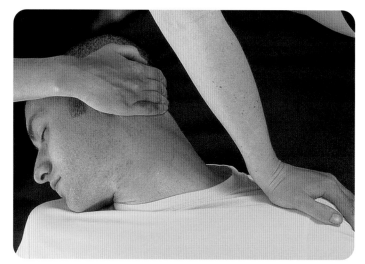

63 Hairwash

Application

- At crown, use thumbs to work down centre Sen line to hairline. Work back to crown and then to hairline again.
- With your fingertips, make small slow circling movements all over scalp, as if washing hair. ▶▶
- Apply pressure, both deep and light.

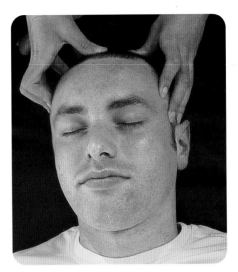

64 Face

Application

- Lightly place your fingers around receiver's jaw line.
- Using both thumbs simultaneously apply TP. Follow the lines of points as shown in diagram, starting at the chin and working up the face. Always work out towards ears. ▶▶
- Moving up, continue following other lines on face with points around eyes finishing at temples. Gently apply TC at end of each line.
- Finish with gentle strokes over face and head in direction of neck to forehead. Follow by gentle strokes of hair.

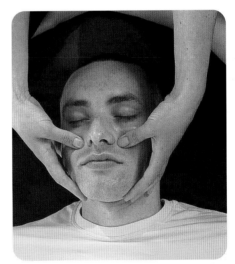

Lines of the face

With a little practice, you will 'feel your way' around the lines of the face without looking.

(Watchpoint)

○ **63 and 64: receiver may need a cushion under their head if the back of the neck has curvature.**

Benefits

Extremely relaxing. Good for draining sinuses and easing headaches. Rejuvenates and stimulates head energy.

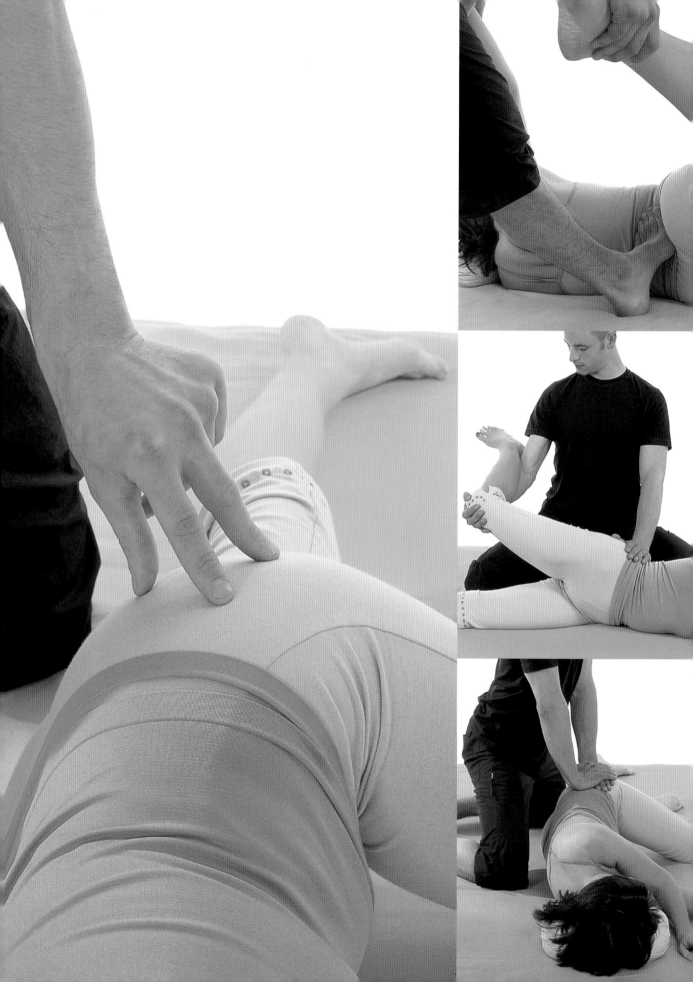

side position

In this position the receiver lies on their side with lower leg extended straight, and upper leg bent in front of them at a right angle to their body. You might like to place a small pillow under their head to make them more comfortable as you work.

65 Inside Leg

Preparation

- Receiver lies with lower leg extended straight, and upper leg bent in front of them at a right angle to body.
- Place a small pillow under their neck for support, if needed.
- Adopt Horse stance behind receiver's extended leg and place one hand at top of receiver's leg, with other hand cupping heel and foot, fingers pointing outwards.

Application

- Inhale, and on the out breath rock on/rock off on to alternate hands to open and stretch Sen lines, in a Hello Stretch. ☒
- PP hands in to knee, PP out to ankle, PP in to knee, then PP down to ankle and foot in Penguin style.
- PP foot with your hands in a loose fist.

66 Inside Sen Lines

Preparation

- Remain in Horse stance (you may also adopt Thai Sitting stance if the receiver is tall and you need to travel up body).

Application

- TP up inside leg line 1 (see page 15) from ankle to knee, and from above knee to the groin, and return keeping Penguin motion. Make sure you are raised enough to deliver TP at perpendicular angle. ▶▶
- TP up line 2 as for line 1 and return.
- TP up line 3 as for others and return.
- Finish with alternate PP up and down leg to close Sen lines.

67 Outside Leg

Preparation
● Adopt an Open Thai Lunge stance, looking up receiver's body. If you are same height as receiver or smaller, adopt Thai Sitting stance between receiver's legs, opening their legs to accommodate.

Application
● Place one hand on hip and one hand on ankle. Rock on/rock off to acknowledge energy lines. ▶▶
● With both hands, PP in to knee, PP out to ankle and hip and PP down to foot.
● TC foot.

68 Outside Sen Lines

● TP line 2 (see page 15) from ankle to hip and return. (Line 1 is difficult to reach with leg positioned like this.)
● TP line 3 and return, making sure that you turn your body, as shown, for upper half of leg, while keeping an upright posture. ▶▶
● Finish with alternate PP up and down leg to integrate both legs.

Watchpoints
○ **Take your time and remember to breathe.**
○ **Maintain Penguin rocking motion during PP and TP, so your own body does not remain static.**
○ **Do not apply TP on varicose veins.**
○ **Do not TP on lower legs for pregnant women.**

Benefits
Opens up energy lines, releasing and unblocking energy. Great for tired legs.

69 Back Thigh

Preparation
- Sit between receiver's legs, with one leg extended (but slightly bent) and placed behind knee of receiver's upper leg. Bend your other leg to keep it out of way.
- Hold foot of receiver's bent leg.

Application
- With foot against back of receiver's thigh, fully stretch your extended leg to compress receiver's thigh, allowing hand supporting their foot to move and extend with stretch. ⩦
- Work in a 1-2-3-2-1 sequence along back of thigh starting at knee.
- Angle your foot respectfully when compressing near groin area.

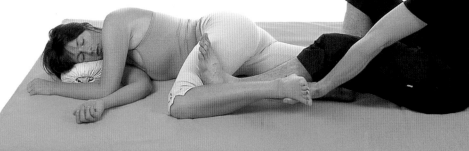

70 Lock Leg

Watchpoints
○ **Make sure angle of compression when working near buttocks is directed towards pelvis. Angle your foot respectfully in this area.**
○ **Work from your hara, not from leg muscles.**

Preparation
- Place both feet against back of receiver's thigh, with one behind knee. You will not move this foot.
- Cross foot of receiver's bent leg across your lower leg, lock, and then hold their heel to keep leg in position.

Application
- Extend your free inside leg and compress receiver's thigh with your foot, starting beside your stationary foot behind the receiver's knee.
- Move along thigh starting at knee in a 1-2-3-2-1 sequence, this time feeling resistance from locked leg. ▸▸

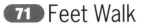 Feet Walk

Preparation
- Sit in same position as for Back Thigh, supporting foot of receiver's bent leg.

Application
- Alternating feet, apply compressions to back of receiver's thigh, 'walking' up and down from behind knee to their buttocks. ⏷

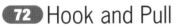 Hook and Pull

Preparation
- Move closer to receiver and place your outer leg on the outside of their bent leg to support their knee.

Application
- Reach across top of their thigh and hook your fingers into Sen line 1 (see page 15). ⏵⏵
- Hook and pull your fingers travelling along the line, working up and down.
- Finish by using Loose Fist to tap out thigh, and wipe down with your hands in a stroking motion.

- Alternate PP up both legs to integrate them, finishing at buttocks ready for next delivery.

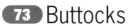

73 Buttocks

Preparation
- Move to Raised Horse stance behind receiver.
- Make sure receiver's bent knee is at a right angle to their waist, and their upper hip is aligned over lower hip.

Application
- Begin with hand on hand clockwise PP circles to whole hip area. ▶▶
- Then apply compression to the three points (see below).
- Follow with TP, keeping thumb perpendicular.
- Close area with (clockwise) PP hand circles.

Watchpoints

- ○ If receiver indicates that certain points are sensitive, still work them as it shows it is needed.
- ○ Take your time with them, and spiral thumb in and out of the points.

Three Points Buttocks

- Points 1 and 2 are at the end of outside Sen line 2.
- Point 3 is at the end of Sen line 3 (where the thumb is in the illustration). ▶▶

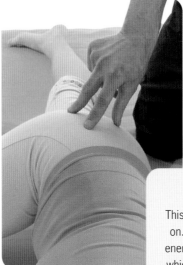

Benefits
This is a powerful area to work on. There are many points of energy release in the buttocks, which, when worked on, affect both legs and lower back, as well as internal organs.

PP and TP Back

Application

● In seated Horse stance, position yourself in centre of your work area, but sitting far enough back from receiver to work with your arms straight with delivery angle perpendicular to back. PP up and down back in laminar groove above spine. Continue up and around trapezius and back again. Moving your body to accommodate. ▸▸

Watchpoints

○ **Keep your own back straight and work from your hara.**
○ **Remember to breathe!**
○ **Do not treat recent slipped disc, but older than three months treat sensitively.**

● Then, placing your thumbs in laminar groove above spine, TP from lower lumbar, up and along to trapezius and back down, using the side to side rocking motion as you do (pressure should be deep and slow). ▸▸
● Finish with PP up to scapular ready for next delivery.

Benefits
Many benefits as points worked on interact with most main organs and major body systems. General relief of tension to lower, middle and upper spine. Great position for late pregnancy (support bent knee with cushion). Old back injuries can benefit.

75 Rotate Shoulder

Preparation

● Kneel beside receiver, facing their head. Kneel close enough that their back is supported against your thigh.
● Lift their upper arm and hook it over your inside arm.
● Clasp both your hands over top of their shoulder.

Application

● Lean back with straight arms and gently pull shoulder towards you, then rotate very slowly three times in each direction, using your bodyweight. ▸▸
● Check receiver is not holding their head off the floor as you pull shoulder toward you but letting it hang and rise naturally with stretch.

76 Trapezius

Preparation

● Bend your inside arm at elbow to raise and support receiver's arm at a right angle, allowing trapezius muscles to relax.

Application

● With fingers of both hands, massage along trapezius line with circular movements. ▸▸

78

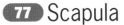 **Scapula**

Preparation
- Hold receiver's shoulder with just one hand now and move back a little to give space to work.
- Gently tip receiver towards you.
- Support your arm by placing your elbow on floor.

Application
- PP around the shoulder blade (scapula).
- Follow with TP, rocking receiver's body towards you and on to your thumb, until you can get your fingers underneath scapula releasing it from back. ▼
- Finish off this section by returning to kneeling position used for Trapezius and generously massage up to neck and scalp, and down again to the trapezius.

Watchpoint

○ **Scapula work is done using receiver's bodyweight rather than your muscle power.**

Benefits
Everybody wants exercises in this section (pages 78–9) done to them!
The Scapula holds a lot of tension and the area between the shoulders is difficult to reach. These techniques free tension, helping headaches and breathing problems, and posture alignment. These exercises also have a knock-on effect in relaxing the diaphragm and digestive system.

78 Stretch Arm

Preparation

- Assume a Thai Lunge stance, making sure your front foot is about parallel with receiver's head.
- Take wrist of receiver's upper arm and hold arm up at right angles to their body.
- Place your other hand, palm down, in their armpit as a listening hand only (see page 20). ▸▸

Application

- Ask receiver to breathe in. On out breath, lift wrist with one hand and gently extend arm over head, stretching in direction away from feet. Return.
- Repeat in a stronger stretch using both hands. ▸▸

Watchpoints

- ○ Do not lower stretch too close to head or floor.
- ○ Some receivers may be very restricted in shoulder joint and so you may need to accommodate by directing arm more in front of body.

Benefits

Opens and stretches body from hip through intercostals to the wrist.

79 Transition Moves

Preparation

● Lower receiver's arm by bringing it round to the front of their body in a flowing circle, and back towards you. ▶▶

● Ensure you are balanced in your position as delivery of this movement will not be as effective if you are not.

Application

● As you bring arm back towards you, lean back and stretch it to open up receiver's body. ▶▶

Watchpoint

○ If receiver lacks flexibility in frontal pectoral muscles, you will need to pull them over more, ready for next move.

81

80 Inside Arm

Preparation

- In extended Thai stance, kneel back on your lower leg.
- Rest receiver's arm across your thigh, holding their wrist on your raised leg. ▸▸
- You may need to move your knee higher up receiver's arm during delivery.

Watchpoint

- ◯ If receiver lacks flexibility, to make them comfortable turn them completely over on to back and work as in supine section for arms.

81 Inside Sen Line

Application

- PP in to elbow, PP out, PP in and PP down to wrist and hand.
- TP along the central inside Sen line, from wrist to shoulder, travelling between biceps and bone on upper arm. ▸▸
- Close with alternate PP up and down arm.

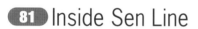

82 Outside Arm

Preparation
● Change your position to Horse stance behind receiver.
● Place receiver's arm against their side.

Application
● With one hand on their shoulder, and another at their wrist, ask receiver to breathe in. On out breath, Hello Stretch the arm. Slowly rock on/rock off, using your bodyweight, pressing your hands away from you. ▶▶
● Follow this with PP in to elbow, PP out, PP in and down the arm.

Watchpoint
○ **If receiver has asthma, do not lean your bodyweight too heavily in 82.**

83 Outside Sen Line

Application
● Now TP central outside sen line of arm, following same sequence as for TP on the inside arm. ▶▶
● Close with alternate PP up and down arm.

Benefits
Opening Sen lines in arm releases a lot of held tension. It is more powerful than it seems, so indulge in it.

84 Hand Sequence

Preparation
● Move your position to Thai Sitting.
● Receiver's arm should still be lying along their side.
● Rotate their hand so palm is facing you, the back of their elbow facing upwards, and their hand supported in yours. ⯯

Application
● The following hand sequence starts with breaking bread (see page 62) followed by random TP, then moves 54–8. Follow same detail as in Supine sequence (see pages 63–5).

85 Transition

● Keeping hold of receiver's hand, bring yourself to a Half Kneeling position level with their shoulder.
● Holding upper arm with one hand, bend arm over towards their head, supporting elbow at all times.
● Place your palm against theirs to guide the hand down. ▶▶
● Place their hand against side of their head, keeping elbow up. The fingertips should be pointing down and round the back of their head, not up over their ears.

86 Stretch Hip to Armpit

Preparation
- Move into a more Open Lunge stance.
- Place one hand on receiver's elbow and other on their hip.

Application
- Ask receiver to breathe in. On out breath stretch elbow and hip away from each other, lifting elbow upwards. ⤓

Watchpoint
○ **Be careful not to stretch delicate skin above elbow in 86 and 87.**

87 Open Intercostals

Application
- With one hand holding elbow to support arm, use the outer hand to lift and stretch arm by lunging in direction away from feet. Apply in a 1-2-3-2-1 sequence from armpit to elbow. ▶▶
- Gently massage triceps.
- Release, and shake arm.

Benefits
Opens intercostals and waist area, armpit and chest.

88 Kneeling Half Locust

Preparation

- Move your position back to kneeling behind receiver's extended leg, but on raised toes.
- Taking ankle of their bent leg, draw it back towards you. ▶▶

- Place your upper hand on receiver's hip to steady their body.
- Cradle leg on your forearm, supporting it with a hand under their knee. ▶▶
- Now place your knee of the leg closest to receiver's head in receiver's sacrum, but do not press into it (see Application 1 photograph, opposite).

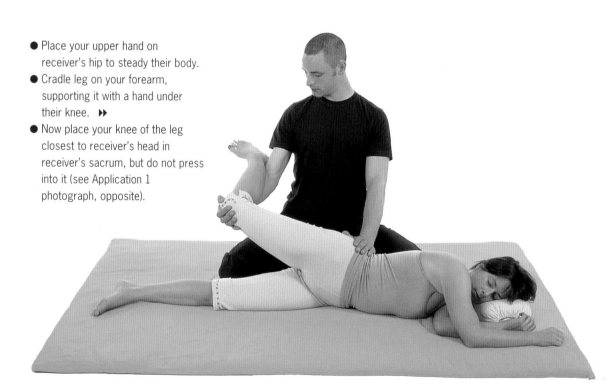

Watchpoints

- It is important to position yourself high enough up receiver's body from beginning to allow a good stretch of front thigh.
- Lean back slightly. Always pull receiver's leg towards your knee.
- Ask receiver for feedback, especially when they have reached maximum stretch.
- Move slowly.

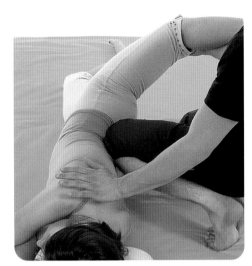

Application 1

- With knee on the lower back/sacrum, gently pull receiver's leg towards you, stretching receiver's front thigh. ◀◀

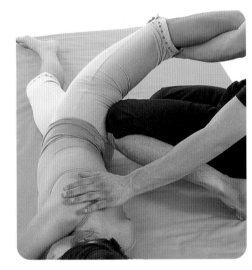

Application 2

- Move same knee down to centre of buttock and again gently pull leg towards you. ◀◀

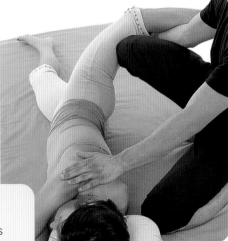

Application 3

- Change to your other knee for next application.
- Move your knee (the one closest to receiver's feet) down to the upper thigh and pull the leg back again.
- Move your knee to mid-thigh and repeat action. ◀◀
- Gently tap out, with hand from receiver's shoulder, using loose fist, along receiver's front thigh, and then smooth down using palm.
- Replace receiver's leg on floor as in 87.

Benefits

Stretches the front thighs and hip flexors. Benefits the large and small intestine.

89 Half Locust Standing

Preparation

● Come to standing position and take hold of ankle of receiver's bent leg, and gently draw it towards you from floor position. Then take hold of their uppermost arm by the wrist, and ask receiver to hold your wrist. Place yourself opposite receiver's waist. Do not lean forward, and keep a straight back by bending your supporting knee.

● Keep both raised leg and arm loose and relaxed.

● Place one foot (heel on the floor) in lowest part of back, making sure ball of the foot is just above spine, supporting it. ▶▶

Watchpoints

○ Be careful not to overstretch arm. Main focus is on leg stretch.

○ Receiver's leg should be drawn towards your lower body, not towards the ceiling.

Application

● Ask receiver to breathe in. On out breath, gently pull up and back on their arm and leg in a seesaw motion, making sure leg lifts more than arm. Ask receiver when maximum stretch is attained. ▶▶

● Replace leg slowly and carefully.

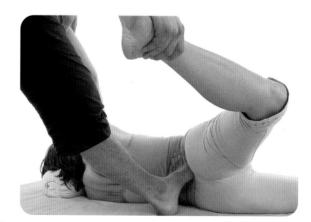

Benefits

Strong stretch travelling from knee through thigh, hip, large intestine to solar plexus.

90 Lifting Cross Twist

Preparation
- Place receiver back in to position shown in 65.
- Place one foot between their legs, behind knee of the bent leg, with other outside their hip. Make sure you feel centred in this position and your feet are parallel. Bend your knees into a squat to prepare for lift using a straight back.
- Hold wrist of the receiver's lower arm, and ask them to hold yours. ▶▶

Application
- Ask receiver to inhale.
- On out breath, very, very slowly pull arm up towards you, bringing receiver's upper body with it. ▶▶
- Lower the body very slowly so vertebrae sink back into position, especially slowly towards the end.
- Raise and lower the receiver three times, each time lifting a little higher. Ask receiver for feedback for maximum stretch.
- PP the lower back.
- **Repeat from move 65 on other side**.

Watchpoints
- ○ **Make sure receiver's head and shoulders are relaxed.**
- ○ **It is essential to work extremely slowly to maximize benefit.**
- ○ **88–90 can be demanding on receiver's lower back. When practising, please be aware of this and apply PP in circular motion.**
- ○ **Do not do this if receiver has recently slipped a disc.**

Benefits
The cross-diagonal twist of the spine really opens up the area between the shoulders, especially if done slowly. Loosens lower back.

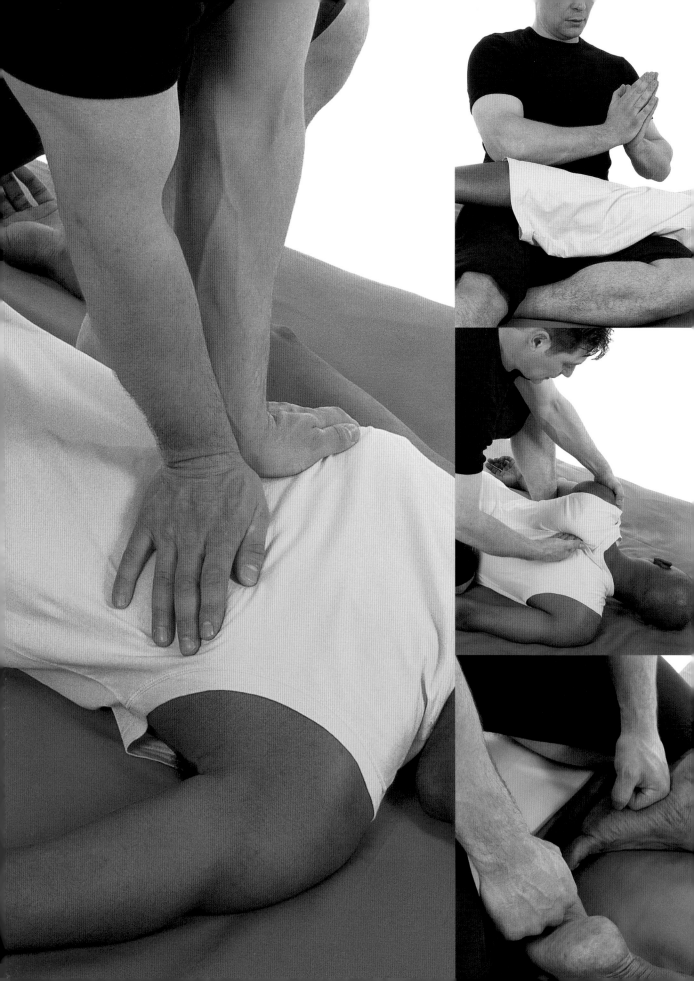

prone position

In the prone position the receiver lies on their front. Some of the moves are quite demanding, so keep checking with the receiver that they are comfortable and provide a cushion for support if required. At the end of this section you will find transition moves for manoeuvring the receiver from one position to another.

91 Hello Legs

Preparation
● Ask receiver to lie on their stomach, with their legs open, hands by sides and head to one side.
● Adopt Kneeling stance.

Application
● To warm up feet and legs, apply loose fist technique to feet (see below) just to say 'hello' and then apply alternate PP up and down back of both legs following centre Sen line from ankles to crease line at buttocks. ⍖

Watchpoints

○ Apply light to medium pressure on calves. Do not PP back of knees. Apply firmer pressure to back of the thighs.

○ Receiver may need a cushion under their stomach if they have lower back problems, or under their chest if their neck is uncomfortable.

○ While working on their back, at intervals ask them to turn their head to other side to prevent tension gathering in one side of neck.

○ Make sure your body weight is applied perpendicularly when travelling along Sen lines.

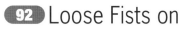

92 Loose Fists on Feet

Application
● Apply Loose Fists technique using alternate presses on sole of each foot, rocking your body in Penguin motion. Pressure can be firm and last up to a minute. ▸▸

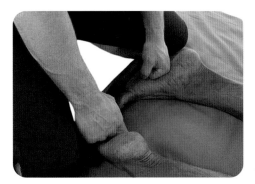

93 Knees to Feet

Application
- Supporting yourself with your hands, kneel in medial arches of soles of feet and rock from side to side in Penguin style applying alternate presses to each foot. ▶▶
- Finish with Loose Fists to close.

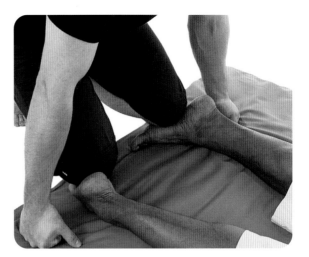

Watchpoints

○ Make sure you have checked whether receiver has arthritis in toes or gout. Either condition would prevent you applying firm pressure, especially for 93.

○ In 93, do not travel too high towards the heel of the instep.

94 Centre Sen Line

Application
- TP using both hands simultaneously up and down centre Sen line. ▶▶

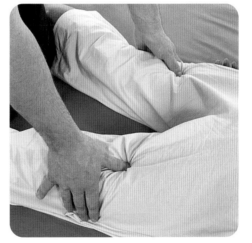

Benefits
Centre Sen line on back of leg is powerful and similar to bladder meridian in the Chinese system. Releasing energy along this line is very nurturing for both legs and feet, especially if they are tired and overworked.
Opening up points on foot starts the stimulation of the Sen lines.

Watchpoints

○ Make sure your body weight is applied perpendicularly when travelling along Sen lines.

○ When applying TP there is a sensitive point just below the calf muscle where you should lighten pressure.

○ Avoid TP if the receiver has varicose veins.

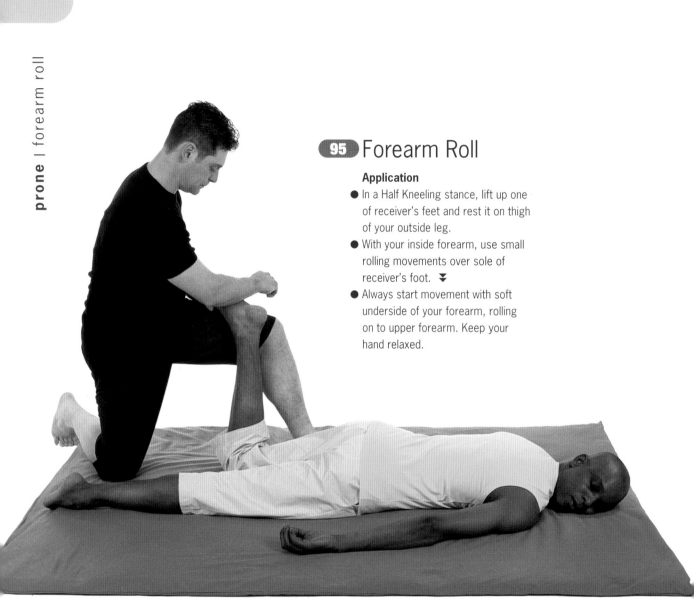

95 Forearm Roll

Application

- In a Half Kneeling stance, lift up one of receiver's feet and rest it on thigh of your outside leg.
- With your inside forearm, use small rolling movements over sole of receiver's foot. ⌄
- Always start movement with soft underside of your forearm, rolling on to upper forearm. Keep your hand relaxed.

Watchpoint

○ Check with the receiver that their lower back is comfortable throughout moves 95 and 96.

96 Six Points

Application
- Hold receiver's toes down in a flexed position.
- Using your elbow, compress the six points of the foot (see page 30). Sink slowly into each point in order, and come out gently releasing each point by dropping your forearm forwards, rather than lifting your elbow off abruptly. ▶▶
- Repeat and finish with a Forearm Roll to close.

97 Five Lines

Application
- Kneel and rest receiver's foot on your thigh. TP the five lines of the foot (see page 31). ⤓
- Caterpillar along the toes.
- Finish by rotating and pressing foot downwards to stretch the Achilles tendon.
- **Repeat 95–7 on other foot.**
- Use Forearm Roll to close points.

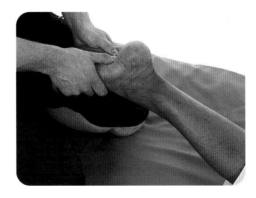

Watchpoints

- ○ **For a deeper effect when using your elbow on the six points, keep receiver's foot flexed. However, if this is too strong, relax the flex.**
- ○ **Sink in slowly with your elbow – especially on points 4, 5 and 6.**

98 Ankle Stretch

Application

- Adopt raised kneeling position and with your hands cupping receiver's toes, slowly push their feet towards their buttocks. ▶▶
- **Repeat twice.**

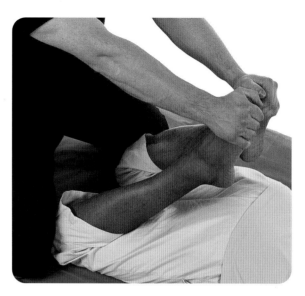

99 Cross Feet

Application

- Now open receiver's knees slightly and cross one foot over other.
- Supporting and holding feet together, press them towards buttocks twice. ▶▶
- **Reverse feet and repeat.**

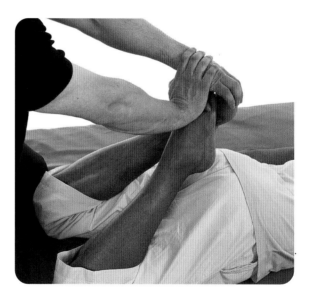

(Watchpoints)

- ○ **98 and 99: it is important to check with the receiver that their lower back is comfortable throughout.**
- ○ **Do not compress too long or too hard.**

Benefit

Front leg stretch from toes to knee and up thigh.

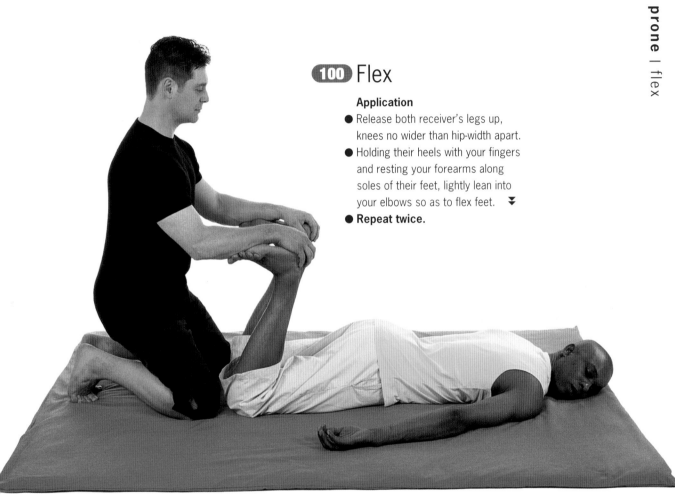

100 Flex

Application

● Release both receiver's legs up,
  knees no wider than hip-width apart.
● Holding their heels with your fingers
  and resting your forearms along
  soles of their feet, lightly lean into
  your elbows so as to flex feet. ⍖
● **Repeat twice.**

97

101 Bent Leg

Preparation

● In a Half Kneeling stance, lift receiver's nearest leg, moving the knee wider, and cross it over their other leg. Place foot of nearest leg behind knee of other leg.

● Bend other leg up and push it gently towards buttocks, locking receiver's foot in place.

Application

● Gently PP buttock and upper thigh of 'crossed over' leg, gently leaning into lunge to apply compression. Use a 1-2-3-2-1 sequence, applying strongest compression at buttock. ⍗

102 Transfer move

● Still holding extended leg up, and keeping the other leg crossed over, transfer your raised knee to the floor as in Horse stance, placing it in line with the receiver's waist. ▸▸

103 Test Stretch

Application
- Holding raised foot with both hands, inside hand on heel, pull it up towards you. ▸▸
- This prepares the body for the next movement and allows you to gauge how far receiver can be stretched in this position.

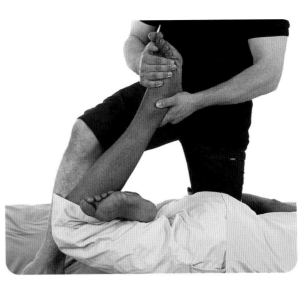

104 Kneeling Half Locust

Preparation
- Still in same position, slide your outside hand to cup receiver's knee, placing foot under your armpit. Place palm of your inside hand on their lower back to support it firmly.

Application
- By leaning back into supporting hand, gently pull knee up towards you as far as is comfortable for receiver, and slowly bring leg back down. ▸▸
- Repeat three times, each time asking receiver how far you can take them into stretch.

Watchpoint

○ **Not to be used on receivers who have had hip or knee replacements.**

Benefits
Kneeling Half Locust is the most powerful of Locust positions, with the added benefit of lower back being supported, and giver, therefore, having good control of movement. Stretches up through front thigh, hip flexor, lower abdomen, and hara to diaphragm.

105 Roll Back

Preparation
- Unfold and straighten receiver's legs and gently slide your own leg under receiver's far leg. Sit sideways to the body, as close to hips as possible, both of your legs bent.
- Receiver's leg should rest across your thigh.
- Hold receiver's ankle with one hand and place your other hand in their lower back, ready for a Forearm Roll.

Application
- Roll arm over lower and middle back, concentrating on the lower back. ⩔

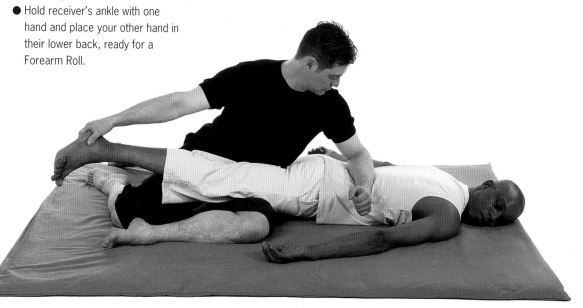

106 Hello Leg Stretch

Application
- Extend your outside leg in front of you, to allow you to sit square.
- Keeping lower hand on receiver's heel, place your other hand in crease of their thigh and buttock.
- Breathe in, and stretch leg through compression, directing your stretch away from centre. ▸▸

Watchpoint

○ Make sure receiver's thigh is well placed on your leg, and that it is not resting 'bone to bone'.

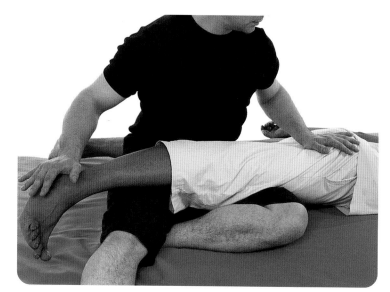

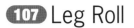 107 Leg Roll

Application

- Use both forearms to roll out along the calf as well as the thigh simultaneously.

- Start with both arms at receiver's knee. Roll out to ankle and buttock and back in to knee, and then slide arms out and off while compressing the leg. ⩣

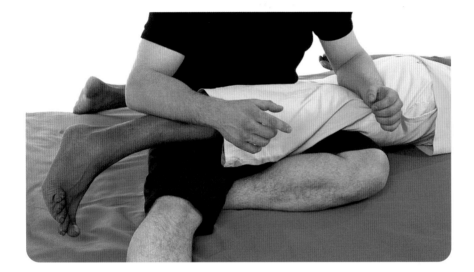

108 Prayerchop

Application

- Finally, relax leg by Prayerchopping down and up buttocks, back of the thigh and calf, but not over knee. ⩣

- **Repeat on other leg from 105–8.**
- Close this leg section with alternate PP up and down back of legs and feet to integrate.

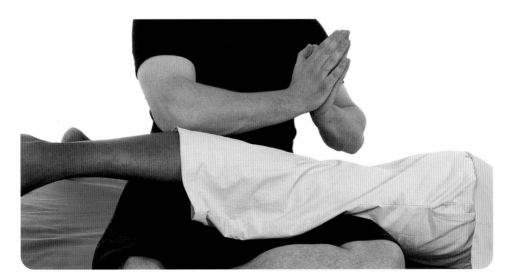

109 PP Sacrum

Preparation
- With receiver's legs extended straight on mat, adopt Thai Lunge position straddling their buttocks.
- Place your palms at base of spine, over sacrum, with heels of your hands centre-sacrum, your fingers pointing outwards in the Butterfly hand position. ▶▶
- Take your time to PP this area.
- Ask receiver to breathe in before each application of PP. Synchronize your breathing with receiver.

Watchpoints
- ○ Ask receiver to turn head to allow neck to stretch and relax on both sides.
- ○ Do not travel your stance up the body while applying the pressure.
- ○ Before starting, check if receiver's back and neck are comfortable; if not they may require a pillow.
- ○ Do not apply PP on recently slipped discs.

Benefits
The slow deep pressure over the sacrum and lumbar region helps to relieve lower back strain.

The points either side of spine are important as they are related to nearly all parts of the body. Because we are upright most of the time, stress and strain easily accumulates here, and the pull of gravity does not help to ease situation.

It also helps to redress a left side/right side imbalance.

110 Butterfly Compression

Preparation

- Place hands in butterfly position over lower lumbar region with heels of hands lying on respective sides of laminar groove.
- Ask receiver to breathe in before each application of PP or TP. Synchronize your breathing with receiver.

Application

- On out breath, do simultaneous PP from the lower lumbar up the spine, taking care not to press down too hard around the kidney area, and only up to the area between the shoulder blades. ▶▶
- Keep angle of delivery perpendicular by moving your body as well as your arms up receiver's body.
- Work back down with alternate PP.

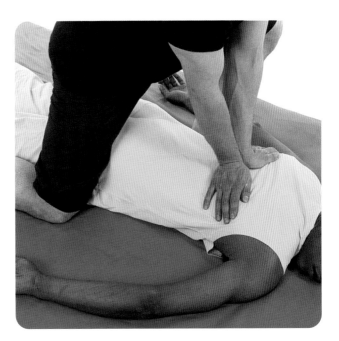

111 Thumb Press

Application

- Work up and down spine, this time using TP in the laminar groove either side of spine, keeping your delivery perpendicular, applying both thumbs simultaneously. ▶▶
- Finish with alternate PP up and down back again to close.

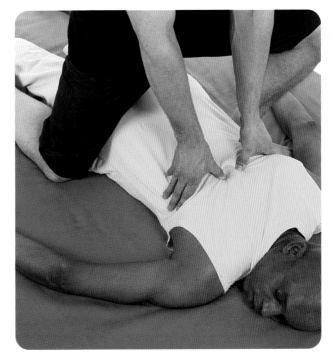

112 Half Kneeling Bow

Preparation
- There are two ways to perform this movement. Most people prefer the Half Kneeling position.
- Adopt a Half Kneeling stance over receiver's back, level with their waist.

Application
- Bending forwards, hold receiver's shoulders. Ask them to breathe in.
- On out breath pull receiver's shoulders back. ▸▸
- Release receiver back to mat slowly, and repeat twice.

Watchpoints
- Done slowly, this movement is usually achievable by all.
- Always ask receiver how far back you can pull them.

113 Seated Bow

Preparation
- Lift both receiver's feet up.
- Place your buttocks on the soles of their feet, with your feet placed near receiver's waist so as to give you leverage.
- Lift receiver's arms up and place them on your thighs. Receiver's ability to do this will depend on their flexibility and arm length. Alternatively, place arms along receiver's body inside your legs.

Application
- Hold their shoulders and pull back in same way as in Half Kneeling position. Repeat twice. ▾
- Try to keep a straight back, drawing your power from your hara.

Benefits
Good for opening chest and bringing flexibility to lower and middle back.

Watchpoint
- The Seated Bow requires flexible pectoral muscles.

114 Scapula

Preparation
- Adopt Half Kneeling stance over receiver's lower back.
- Place one palm under receiver's shoulder and raise it up and inwards a little.
- Make sure receiver's head is facing in the direction of worked shoulder.

Application
- With your other hand PP around shoulder blade (scapula), gently rocking receiver's shoulder towards your working hand.
- Hold your hand so that your thumb is pointing in under edge of shoulder blade. ⍗
- TP around entire area from top to bottom and back, pulling shoulder back on to your thumb, rather than pushing thumb in underneath.

Watchpoints
○ **Do not lean too far over receiver or it will be you that needs treatment!**
○ **Draw your strength from your hara and buttocks.**
○ **If receiver's shoulder is tense, circle whole shoulder a few times to get it to 'let go'.**
○ **Receiver's head and neck need to be comfortable. Some people have difficulty turning their head to a particular side, so ask them to turn their head slowly.**

- Turn your hand over and this time work shoulder blade from top to bottom and back, this time pulling it back on to your fingers. ▶▶
- Finish off with PP around receiver's shoulder blade.
- Repeat on other side, changing to your other leg.

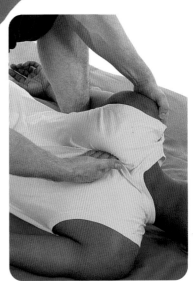

Benefit
Everyone loves having this area worked on because it holds so much tension, so take your time and indulge receiver.

105

115 Cobra 1

Preparation
● Place your knees at centre of receiver's buttocks. Ask receiver to grasp your wrists, as you grasp theirs.

Application
● Ask receiver to breathe in, and on out breath, lean back and gently lift. Ensure they are not holding themselves up. ▸▸
● Lower them slowly and ask them to change head to other side.

● Repeat with your knees between mid-buttock and crease line and again just below crease line of buttock and thigh.
● Ask receiver to let you know when they have reached their maximum stretch.
● Finish with alternate PP up and down the back, ready for Cobra 2.

116 Cobra 2

Preparation
● Place your knees on Point 3.
● Walk your hands up to between receiver's shoulder blades, your bottom sitting on your heels, arms stretched out and relaxed – placed at the highest raised part of thoracic, roughly between shoulder blades.

Application
● Ask receiver to inhale, and on out breath slide your upper body forward with arms bent then lift up on to straight arms into Cobra pose. ▸▸
● Return in reverse order.

Benefits
Stretches and opens front torso and opens chest. Helps flexibility of back.

Watchpoints
○ **Do not place your hands too high as they will slide into receiver's neck during application.**
○ **Do not hold Cobra 2 for more than 3–5 seconds.**
○ **Asthmatics may find the compression rather uncomfortable.**

Benefits
Releases tension between shoulders and provides lung compression.

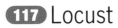 Locust

Preparation
● Stand between receiver's knees and lift their legs up by the feet, as if you were holding a wheelbarrow, checking that their legs are relaxed at all times.
● Place foot on receiver's lower back, turning it so it is parallel to your body.
● Check receiver's legs are relaxed by observing the knees and buttocks.

Application
● As receiver exhales, carefully lift their legs higher.
● There are two techniques for this move. Most people prefer No. 1.
  1 Place foot as support only and concentrate on the 'lift'. ▸▸
  or
  2 Compress by gently leaning into foot in the lower back. Application angle is perpendicular to floor.
● Lower legs a little and repeat extended lift.

(**Watchpoint**)

○ **Make sure anchor foot is turned out to facilitate application stability.**

118 Half Locust

Preparation
● Stand on one side of receiver, anchor leg between waist and armpit not too close to receiver.
● Hold wrist of arm nearest to you (and ask receiver to hold yours) and ankle of the leg farthest from you.
● Place your foot at receiver's lower back.
● Check receiver's limbs are relaxed.

Application
● Without pressing your foot into waist, first draw their leg towards you then release. Next stretch and release the arm. Repeat this a few times, creating a subtle see-saw motion. ◂◂
● Finish by gently stretching both arm and leg together, with more stretch directed to leg. Ask receiver to let you know when they have reached maximum stretch.
● Repeat on other side.

119 Cross Stretch

Preparation
- Adopt Half Kneeling stance on one side of receiver.
- Place one hand on shoulder blade and with other cup the opposite hip bone, fingers pointing outwards.

Application
- Ask receiver to inhale, and on out breath lean in with your weight and compress with both hands as if you were pushing them away from the centre, creating a cross stretch. ◀◀
- **Repeat**.

Watchpoint
○ **Your body needs to be placed centrally over work area.**

- Move hands to other shoulder and hip and repeat the above. ⤓
- Finish by circling palms over back. Stroke down area.

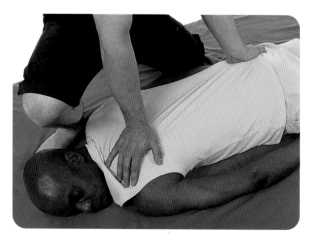

Benefit
Relaxes and settles the torso.

108

120 Hamstring Crunch

Preparation

- Ask receiver to turn over very slowly on to their back.
- Raise their legs and place their feet against your chest, or beside your waist. Place your feet around their buttocks. Where they can place their feet will depend on your relative body sizes.
- Bend your legs slightly.
- Grasp each other's wrists. ▸▸

Application

- Breathe in together and on out breath, pull receiver up towards you, drawing your elbows up to facilitate maximum stretch of the hamstrings. Make sure receiver's bottom stays on ground. You only want to raise their upper body.
- **Repeat three times.**
- Finish by lowering receiver to floor ready for next move.

Benefits

Stretches the backs of the legs (the hamstrings) and opens the lower back.

120 and 121 may be used at any time for releasing lower back and also as transition between positions: prone to seated, supine to seated, side to seated.

121 Crossed Legs

Preparation
- Ask receiver to bend and cross their legs against your slightly bent legs.
- Make sure they are comfortable with no bone lying against bone.
- Grasp each other's wrists. ▸▸

Application
- Breathe in, and on out breath pull receiver's torso up towards their knees, at same time straightening your own. ▸▸
- Repeat twice, then ask receiver to cross their legs the other way and repeat.
- On last move, when receiver's body has been pulled up, bend your legs slightly to facilitate a compression, creating a stronger stretch.
- At this point you may lay them down or bring them to sitting position using Lift Up.

Benefit
Releases lower back.

110

122 Lift Up

Application

- If you wish them to be seated, take a few steps back until you have pulled them up into a sitting position.
- Support receiver's hands for a few seconds until they feel centred as this simple lift creates quite an uplifting feeling. ▶▶

Watchpoint

○ Some receivers may feel a little giddy when first pulled upright, but this quickly settles into a pleasant, light feeling.

Benefit

Prepares the receiver in a safe way for coming up into the sitting position.

111

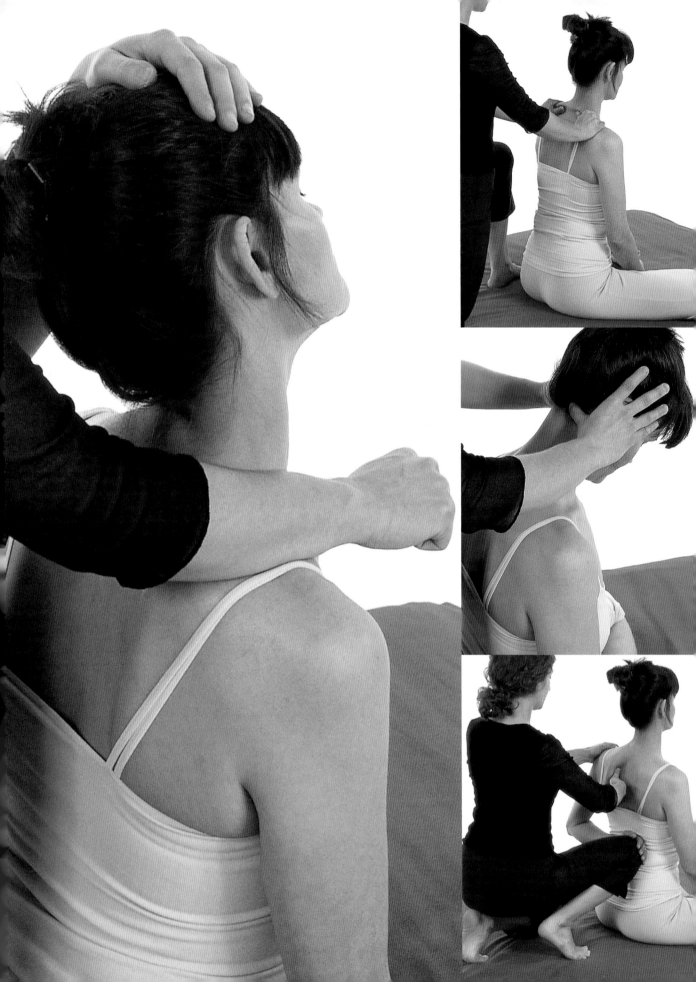

seated position

The receiver sits on a mat on the floor with their legs crossed. If the receiver is unable to sit cross legged, most of these exercises can be adapted so that the receiver can sit on a stool, or sit facing the back of a dining chair.

123 Shoulder Compression

Preparation
- With a meditative mind, step in and stand behind receiver with your feet turned out and legs supporting receiver's back.

Application
- With your fingers pointing down receiver's back, ask receiver to breathe in. On out breath, apply three double palm compressions.
- Work out from the neck to edges of shoulders. ⤓

Watchpoint

- Receiver's back must be aligned as straight as possible, but relaxed, **BEFORE** you start.

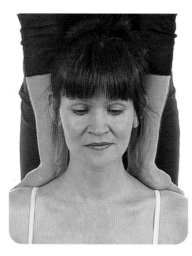

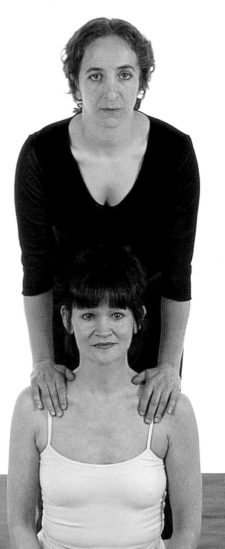

- Reverse your hands so that your fingers are pointing down the chest. Return back to the neck, repeating palm compressions. ▶▶

Benefits
Provides a wonderful tension release to shoulders, neck and breathing.

124 Shoulders

Preparation
● Adopt Half Kneeling stance.

Application
● Gently knead the trapezius with heel of alternate hands, like a cat kneads with its paws. ▸▸

Watchpoint

○ Take care when massaging that your fingers do not pinch the front of the shoulders. Focus is on the thumbs on the back of trapezius and shoulders.

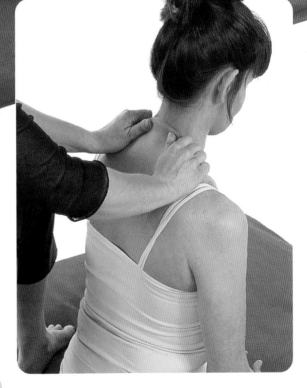

● Then massage the trapezius with your thumbs, using a circular squeezing motion. ▸▸

Benefits
Deeper release of tension.
Indulge!

125 Back Flexor

Preparation

- Ask receiver to support themselves by leaning forwards and placing their hands in front of them on mat, head down, keeping arms straight at all times.
- Adopt Half Kneeling stance far enough away from receiver so that you can keep your arms straight.
- Start by placing your hands between shoulder blades (mid-thoracic) ready to give Butterfly double palm compressions down the back.
- Ask receiver to breathe in and out. ▶▶

Application

- On out breath, give compression by leaning into a deeper lunge. Receiver and giver bring their heads up simultaneously. Keep your arms straight. ▶▶
- Release, inhale, drop your heads again, place your hands in a lower position and repeat.
- Repeat this three or four times, moving down to just below waist.
- Finish by walking your hands back up using alternate PP.

Benefits

Loosens up the area all along spine.
Opens up energy points and releases blockages.

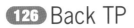 **Back TP**

Application

● TP both thumbs simultaneously down laminar groove on either side of the spine, taking your time and breathing together with the receiver. Move your thumbs down the back about 2.5 cm (1 inch) at a time. ▸▸

Watchpoints

○ **Keep your arms straight.**
○ **Keep your back as straight as possible.**

● You will need to move farther from receiver as you progress down spine to allow arms to stay straight and for correct angle of delivery. ▸▸
● Use alternate PP to walk back up spine, keeping your fingers pointing out to sides.

117

127 Scapular

Preparation

- Return receiver to sitting upright again. Adopt Half Kneeling stance.
- Place receiver's hand behind their back, palm facing outwards, and support it in position with your opposite knee. Bring your knee to their hand, not their hand to your knee.
- Support shoulder of the side you are working on with outside hand.

Application

- With your inside hand PP around edge of the shoulder blade (scapula), working down and then up, drawing shoulder to your hand in a slight rocking motion.
- TP holding your thumb so that it points in and underneath shoulder blade. ⧩
- Pull shoulder back a little so that it rolls back on to your thumb.
- Finish with PP around area, keeping rocking motion going throughout.
- Repeat on other scapular, changing over to your other knee.

Benefits

Working scapular in this position allows receiver freedom of movement and good access to giver.

128 Forearm Roll

Preparation
- Retain Half Kneeling position.
- Gently and slowly place your palm over top of receiver's head, and tilt it to one side.

Application
- Apply a forearm roll to receiver's shoulder, working out to edge of shoulder and back.
- Start roll with your fist loose – palm down, rolling to palm up. ▸▸
- **Repeat on other side.**

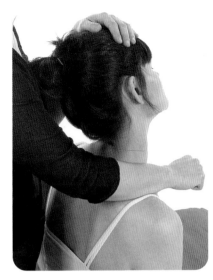

Watchpoints

- ○ Take care not to rest weight on receiver's head.
- ○ Receiver needs to sit up straight.
- ○ If receiver's head is dropped too low in 129 and 130, muscles will be too stretched to work on.

129 Nutcracker

Preparation
- Ask receiver to lower their head just a little.

Application
- Clasp your hands and warm receiver's neck by squeezing heels of hands firmly together, working up and down neck. ▸▸

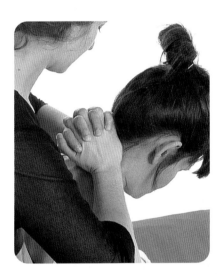

130 Ice Pick

Preparation
- Keep your hands clasped in same position. Lift your elbows.
- Place your thumbs on neck, in laminar grooves on either side of spine.

Application
- Starting at top of the neck, work your thumbs down and up grooves. (Drop and lift your elbows a little to allow thumbs to come together in the proper action.) ▸▸
- **Finish by repeating 129.**

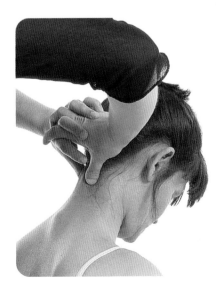

Benefit
Wonderful release of neck tension.

131 Cervical Neck Massage

Preparation
- Move Half Kneeling stance around to side of receiver.
- Hold receiver's head with one hand to steady them. Warm up neck by squeezing and kneading it gently.

Application
- Apply TP on nearside of spine gently but firmly pushing muscle tissue towards you and away from receiver's spine. Repeat on the other side. Take your time with this and indulge the receiver. ▸▸

Watchpoint
○ Check receiver has a floppy head! If 'holding', their neck muscles will be tense and unreceptive.

132 Occipital Ridge

Preparation
- Place thumbs of both hands on occipital ridge, (bottom of the skull), spreading your fingers on each side of head to add stability.

Application
- TP out, travelling along base of skull to ears and back in again, circling each point for a few seconds. ▸▸

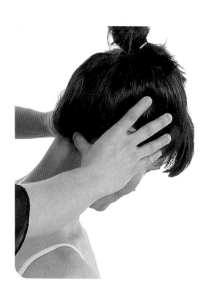

Watchpoint
○ Some of these points may be tender to touch. Be sensitive.

133 Scalp

Application

- Place both hands on receiver's head. Make small circles into and over the scalp. Move slowly. ▶▶
- Now circle from centre of occipital ridge up to crown, in an up-down-up sequence.
- Finish using a lighter touch over scalp, and then comb through receiver's hair with fingers to relax even more.

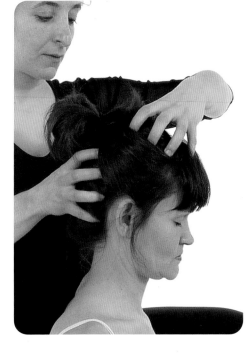

134 Face

Preparation

- Rest receiver's head against your chest so they can relax their neck.

Application

- With your fingertips, make light delicate circles using pad of third finger over all the points shown on the face diagram (see page 69). ▶▶
- To finish, very lightly feather-stoke face and then run your fingers through hair or stroke.

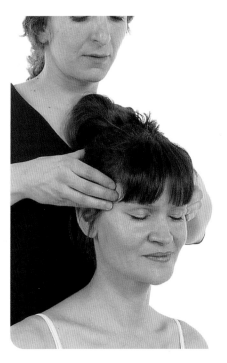

Benefits

This is seriously relaxing and is great for headaches, mental fatigue and stress.

135 Angel Stretch

Preparation
- Change your supporting leg if you feel tired or uncomfortable.
- The giver may also stand behind receiver, their forearms cupping receiver's elbows from over the top. Giver's legs are close to receiver, supporting their back.
- Ask receiver to clasp their hands behind their head.

Application
- Be close enough to support receiver's back, cup their elbows, and ask them to breathe in. On out breath gently draw them towards you until they are at a comfortable full stretch. Ask receiver for feedback during stretch. Release and repeat. ▶▶

Benefits
Opens chest.
Stretches pectorals, armpits and upper arms.
Helps release mid-thoracic in back, aiding flow of energy up and down spine.

Watchpoint
○ **Take care if receiver has had a shoulder injury.**

136 Seated Cross Twist

Preparation

- Slide both of your hands under receiver's arms and gently hold forearms near wrist.
- Move around to side of receiver.
- Your supporting knee should be placed on floor near receiver's buttock.
- Lightly place your other knee on receiver's thigh, starting on upper part of thigh, near hip.
- Do not let receiver's body bend forwards.
- If receiver is not very flexible in pectorals or is much smaller than you, use same position as for the Angel Stretch.

Application

- Breathe in, and on out breath, twist receiver gently round towards you, away from held leg, then return to starting position.
- Move your knee hold from hip to knee in a 1-2-3-2-1 sequence. Position 3 near knee will be the strongest. ▶▶
- Repeat on other side.

Benefits

Stretches and opens the body diagonally, across the spine. Opens the chest and pectorals. Great for lower back.

Watchpoints

- Do not kneel on receiver's knee. Your weight should be supported by you at all times.
- Pay close attention to receiver when performing this technique. Ask them how they feel, if you are unsure.
- Your knee movement allows varying degrees of diagonal stretch. However, if you find it difficult to apply, place your knee in one position until you feel more confident.

137 Row Boat

Preparation

- Ask receiver to stretch out their legs in front.
- Sit behind receiver with your legs in front of you, close enough that your legs are bent.
- Ask receiver to take hold of your wrists. You hold theirs.
- Place your feet over their shoulder blades.

Application

- Breathe in together and on out breath stretch your legs, gently pushing your feet into the back, at the same time pulling the arms back gently. Release.
- Move down to just under scapular, and on application allow toes to sink under shoulder blades. ⬇
- Repeat a little lower down back, then return.

Watchpoints

- You may need to adjust your distance depending on length of your legs and receiver's arms.
- More emphasis is given to feet pushing into receiver's back than on pulling their arms.

Benefits

Great for opening chest and thoracic vertebrae. Also stretches shoulders and pectoral muscles.

138 Forward Hamstring Stretch

Preparation
● With receiver still sitting with their legs straight in front of them, adopt an Open Thai Lunge stance.
● Ask receiver to relax forwards and place their hands beside their legs on mat.

Application
● Ask receiver to breathe in, and on out breath, apply your bodyweight to double palm compressions, working from the middle to lower back. ⩔
● PP back up using alternate PP.

● To close, bring receiver back to original seated position. You can then do the following techniques which are not shown:
● Percussion, to vitalize focus and energy.
● Prayerchop out along shoulders and down one side of spine (but avoid the kidneys). Prayerchop back up.
● Follow with alternate Loose Fist to trapezius, upper back and shoulders.
● Knead shoulders.
● Finish with three or four stroking movements down back, and out to sides.

Watchpoints
○ Check receiver's head is relaxed and not holding, so stretch may continue through to base of skull and relieve neck.
○ Keep your own arms straight. Work from hara.

Benefits
Opens and stretches back of body from heels to base of skull. Especially good for hamstrings and lower back.

index

list of exercises

acknowledgements

Executive Editor: Jane McIntosh   Senior Editor: Sarah Ford
Senior Designer: Rozelle Bentheim   Designer: Ginny Zeal   Photographer: Peter Pugh Cook
Production Controller: Lucy Woodhead   Indexer: Hilary Bird